CAMBRIDGE LIBRARY COLLECTION

Books of enduring scholarly value

History of Medicine

It is sobering to realise that as recently as the year in which On the Origin of Species was published, learned opinion was that diseases such as typhus and cholera were spread by a 'miasma', and suggestions that doctors should wash their hands before examining patients were greeted with mockery by the profession. The Cambridge Library Collection reissues milestone publications in the history of Western medicine as well as studies of other medical traditions. Its coverage ranges from Galen on anatomical procedures to Florence Nightingale's common-sense advice to nurses, and includes early research into genetics and mental health, colonial reports on tropical diseases, documents on public health and military medicine, and publications on spa culture and medicinal plants.

Lectures on General Nursing

Eva Charlotte Ellis Lückes (1854–1919) was a pioneer of nursing training and friend of Florence Nightingale. In 1880, aged only twenty-six, she became matron of the London Hospital, the largest hospital in England, a post she held until her death. During her time there she improved working conditions for the nurses and trained her own staff, recognising the importance of a knowledge of anatomy and physiology, but never losing sight of the primary duty of a nurse to care for a patient's needs. First published in book form in 1884, these lectures were part of the training for probationers at the London Hospital. Emphasising the importance of attention to detail, the lectures address the practicalities of nursing, covering such topics as the management of infection, caring for sick children, bandaging techniques, and drug administration. Also reissued in this series is Lückes's popular 1886 textbook *Hospital Sisters and their Duties*.

Cambridge University Press has long been a pioneer in the reissuing of out-of-print titles from its own backlist, producing digital reprints of books that are still sought after by scholars and students but could not be reprinted economically using traditional technology. The Cambridge Library Collection extends this activity to a wider range of books which are still of importance to researchers and professionals, either for the source material they contain, or as landmarks in the history of their academic discipline.

Drawing from the world-renowned collections in the Cambridge University Library and other partner libraries, and guided by the advice of experts in each subject area, Cambridge University Press is using state-of-the-art scanning machines in its own Printing House to capture the content of each book selected for inclusion. The files are processed to give a consistently clear, crisp image, and the books finished to the high quality standard for which the Press is recognised around the world. The latest print-on-demand technology ensures that the books will remain available indefinitely, and that orders for single or multiple copies can quickly be supplied.

The Cambridge Library Collection brings back to life books of enduring scholarly value (including out-of-copyright works originally issued by other publishers) across a wide range of disciplines in the humanities and social sciences and in science and technology.

Lectures on General Nursing

*Delivered to the Probationers
of the London Hospital
Training School for Nurses*

Eva C.E. Lückes

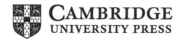

CAMBRIDGE
UNIVERSITY PRESS

CAMBRIDGE UNIVERSITY PRESS

Cambridge, New York, Melbourne, Madrid, Cape Town,
Singapore, São Paolo, Delhi, Mexico City

Published in the United States of America by Cambridge University Press, New York

www.cambridge.org
Information on this title: www.cambridge.org/9781108054270

© in this compilation Cambridge University Press 2012

This edition first published 1884
This digitally printed version 2012

ISBN 978-1-108-05427-0 Paperback

LECTURES ON GENERAL
NURSING

LECTURES

ON

GENERAL NURSING

DELIVERED TO

THE PROBATIONERS OF THE LONDON HOSPITAL

TRAINING SCHOOL FOR NURSES

BY

EVA C. E. LÜCKES

MATRON TO THE LONDON HOSPITAL

LONDON

KEGAN PAUL, TRENCH & CO., 1, PATERNOSTER SQUARE

1884

PREFACE.

DURING a portion of my training as a nurse I was privileged
to attend the lectures to nurses given for several years by
Dr. Allchin at Westminster Hospital. I have frequently
been glad that I was fortunate enough to have the nursing
question at the time when my attention was first turned to
the subject, placed before me from his point of view. I
believe this fact to have been of much service to me, and I
hope by this time to many others, for whose training I have
been, in a measure, responsible.

I am also much indebted to Dr. Allchin for his kind
assistance in preparing the plan of these lectures when I
delivered them for the first time to the probationers of the
London Hospital three or four years ago. It will be obvious
to all that, in adopting to a large extent the classification laid
down by Dr. Allchin, I have not attempted to follow it out on
the technical lines indicated and ably carried out by him in
his own lectures. But, partly from having learnt to regard
the subject originally from his point of view, and partly from
having failed to find elsewhere any other system which

appeared to me equally clear and comprehensive, I have from
the first utilized his classification as a means of conveying in
the most systematic method such information on the general
details of nursing as appears essential for the teaching of
nurses.   At the same time I must not conceal from the
public that for the bulk of the material in these lectures I
alone am responsible.   I am glad, however, to have this
opportunity of gratefully acknowledging my personal obligation to Dr. Allchin.   In compiling these lectures I read many
works connected with the subject, with the view of getting
together as much useful information as possible for the
benefit of those I had to teach.   I have been much helped by
several of these works, and in making use of the valuable
suggestions I have found I have endeavoured, as far as
possible, to acknowledge the source whence they were derived.

So much has already been written on the subject of
nursing, that there is but little scope left for originality, and
my sole object has been to collect as much practical information as possible, and place it before those studying the matter
as simply as I could.

It will be remembered that these lectures only form the
first course of the complete set given every year to probationers training at the London Hospital.   I have confined
myself for the most part to minute details, that are usually
considered almost too trivial to mention, and I believe it is this
fact which chiefly explains the kind appreciation they have
met with from the probationers, and the frequent requests for

their publication. I have felt the more at liberty thus to limit my instructions, from the knowledge that everything I have failed to teach will be more fully and ably set before the probationers in the courses of lectures which regularly follow mine. Mr. Treves' lectures on Elementary Anatomy and Surgical Nursing are complete in themselves, and the same applies to the lectures on Elementary Physiology and Medical Nursing so kindly given by Dr. Sansom. The repetition involved in listening to different lectures much on the same subject can scarcely fail to make the information given more familiar to the hearers, and I heartily share in the gratitude felt by the whole nursing staff for the unwearied kindness and patience with which these gentlemen have been careful to make the theoretical education of the proba tioners of the London Hospital thorough, comprehensive, and complete.

I take this opportunity of mentioning this fact, because I should be sorry for any one reading these lectures to be under the impression that they indicate the limit of the instruction given in this training school for nurses. At the same time, if these lectures contain useful information, I can but hope that their publication will extend the possibilities of such usefulness as they may possess. In the first place, I am hopeful that in this form they may be of service to past, present, and future nurses of the London Hospital; and, in the second place, that other hospital and private nurses may derive some benefit from them.

I am anxious to express my very cordial thanks to all those who have at any time helped me, directly or indirectly, with any hints or suggestions in connection with nursing. I could not have expressed such definite views as I have occasionally ventured to do had they not been derived from the practical knowledge of many accomplished nurses as well as from my own personal experience.

EVA C. E. LÜCKES,

Matron to the London Hospital.

March 3rd, 1884.

CONTENTS.

———◆———

LECTURE I.

LECTURE II.

LECTURE III.

LECTURE IV.

x   CONTENTS.

The following is a list of works on nursing that may be consulted with advantage :—

"A Handbook of Nursing." C. Wood. Cassell, Petter, Galpin, & Co.

"Notes on Nursing." F. Nightingale. Harrison, Pall Mall.

"Handbook for Hospital Sisters." F. Lees. Dalby, Isbister, & Co.

"Handbook for Hospital Nurses." Morrell. Rivington.

"Handbook for Nurses of the Sick." Veitch.

"Handbook of Nursing," published by Lippincott & Co.

"Notes on the Care of the Sick." Brinckman. Palmer.

"Medical Nursing." Dr. Anderson. Maclehose & Sons, Glasgow.

"Manual of Nursing." Cullingworth. J. & A. C. Churchill.

LECTURES ON NURSING.

———◆◇◆———

LECTURE I.

You all know that the cure and care of the sick and injured depend mainly upon doctors and nurses.

The *science* of medicine and the *art* of nursing materially assist each other in their ultimate objects; *i.e.*, of the cure where that is possible, and, failing that, of the alleviation of suffering.

I want you fully to recognize the wide distinction, both in kind and in degree, between the knowledge necessary for a doctor and the knowledge necessary for a nurse, that you may have a clear and definite idea in your minds of what a "trained nurse" should know and be, and that you may not waste time and energy in endeavouring to acquire the sort of information that will not be of real service to you in your own distinct work.

When you reflect for a moment what a complicated machine the human body is, and what a vast amount there is to be learned respecting it, you will not find it difficult to believe that years of study are not sufficient to attain a complete knowledge of it. There is the study of anatomy, which teaches us what the body *is;* *i.e.*, its general structure, size, weight, and so on. The relationship and position of each

B

separate organ, how and of what material each part is made;
—this alone, with the daily advancing discoveries of science,
is an inexhaustible source of study. The same may be said
of physiology, which is the science that teaches us what the
body *does; i.e.*, how the heart beats, for instance, and how the
different organs work. Then the chemical composition of the
body—the various elements of which it is composed, and how
the various tissues are affected by different things. This forms
the third science which is essential to the understanding of
the human body—first, in its healthy condition, and next
under the varied morbid conditions of disease. But when all
this is known, it only becomes the groundwork upon which
the doctor builds his subsequent studies into the nature of
disease, how to find it out, how to prevent it, and how to
cure it.

It is evident that the most studious nurses can only gain
a superficial knowledge of all these subjects, and fortunately
it is not necessary that they should be thoroughly acquainted
with them. But it is essential that you should know those
points in each science that will materially assist you in the
cultivation and understanding of the art of nursing itself.

It is very desirable that you should have a clear idea of
what a doctor is, and what relation you, as nurses, bear to him.
The doctor, when called to a sick person, first turns his
attention to finding out what is the matter. This may be
very obvious, such as a broken leg, an epileptic fit, or an
attack of measles, or it may require a good deal of examining
and questioning on his part. When once he has made a
diagnosis, as it is called, or ascertained in what way the
patient is affected, he proceeds to determine a plan for the
treatment of the case, and, if need be, to prevent any spread
of disease to those about. Up to this point, you as nurses
have no place. In the subsequent conduct of the case, it
will be your part to efficiently carry out the doctor's orders,

and to intelligently and carefully observe, for the purpose of reporting with absolute accuracy, what occurs in the doctor's absence. It is by educating your perceptive faculties in this direction that you may become of such valuable assistance in aiding the cure and alleviation of the sick But important, and very important, as it is that you should be strictly accurate in such points, it is, after all, as agents in administering a system of relief to the patient that you find your place. In the treatment of the case you have your work.

A plan, based upon scientific principles, is laid down by the doctor to himself, and he entrusts much of the carrying out of that plan to you. Hence, at the outset, you see that your work is of no mean order, and that you are placed in a responsible position, requiring intelligence and skill; that, in fact, you are the practisers of an *art*, now acknowledged to be such, and which depends for much of its advancement upon *you*. No doctor can refuse to learn of some matters from a nurse, for he is conscious of her greater familiarity with, and even of her greater aptitude in, many details; but he will most properly resent any interference on her part with those subjects which are within his own sphere. Hence it comes that you have to consider the methods of administering relief. How to make poultices, and how to put them on; not *why* and *when*, that rests with the doctor. How best a patient may be made comfortable in bed, and how that bed may be made; not why he should go to bed, nor how long he should remain there.

Your work as sisters and nurses is neither to rival nor interfere with that of doctors; but in every sense to *help* them. Is not nursing so distinctly a woman's work, chiefly because it is *helping* work, if it is rightly done? This has been, or should be, the characteristic of woman's work from the Creation; so it is by no means taking a lower standard for ourselves to acknowledge this, or rather to aim that it should be so, and I think in working we cannot do better than keep this idea in our minds.

Scrupulously avoid anything which approaches to amateur doctoring, not only for your own sake, but for the sake of the whole nursing profession. It prejudices all who come in contact with it against the education of nurses, and is held in as much contempt by all really accomplished nurses as any other sort of quackery is by duly qualified practitioners.

You must not think, because I am anxious to put you on your guard against those errors which bring so much discredit upon trained nurses, that I am inclined to underrate the importance of your work. On the contrary, I am desirous for you to realize that it ultimately depends not upon the public, but upon *yourselves*, whether you will let yourselves be universally considered efficient helps, and be valued and respected accordingly, or whether you will prove yourselves unworthy and incompetent to fill the satisfactory position which is now open to you.

I want you to think very seriously of the work you have taken up. It is not easy nor insignificant. If you are tempted to fancy so, think of the *power* which rests in your hands. How completely all the doctor's efforts for his patients may be frustrated by careless carrying out, or neglect of his orders, and how terrible the consequences may be! Life may be literally lost, or suffering cruelly increased by ignorant or inefficient nursing. So very much depends upon you that you can scarcely exaggerate the importance of making yourselves in every way fit for the trust which is reposed in you. If, on the other hand, you measure your work by its difficulties, by the patient courage which it demands from you, by the real strength of character which it takes to go on quietly doing the sometimes disagreeable and often wearisome duties which fall to your share day after day, or night after night, as the

case may be, you will not be inclined to say that nursing is
work that "anybody can do."

We hear of people being "born nurses," as though some
favoured mortals came into the world with an instinctive
knowledge of the subject; but experience shows us that this
is not exactly the case. Doubtless some have much greater
natural gifts for nursing than others; but this, like other
arts, such as music or painting, must be carefully cultivated,
studied, and practised, before satisfactory results can be
produced, and the real talent, which some are fortunate
enough to possess, is duly developed.

I would have you set a very high standard before you, and
earnestly resolve that you will not rest satisfied with attaining
anything short of the very best. Your object must be to do
everything connected with your patients in such a manner as
never to give them the least unnecessary pain or discomfort.
It is worth while taking a great deal of trouble over quite
a small detail—and to take trouble is not necessarily to take
time, for to be gentle as well as quick is a habit gained by
proper training—if by so doing you can cause less suffering;
and the knowledge that you are able to do this, is one of the
greatest pleasures you will derive from becoming skilful.

Unless you are prepared to be very patient and painstaking over all the innumerable "little things," your work
will never be thoroughly "trustworthy," and consequently
no credit to yourselves or others. You must endeavour to
learn and to do as *much* as you possibly can, and not rest
contented with "as little."

You have chosen a profession in which there is simply no
limit to the good you can do. Strive to see what your
opportunities are, and then take care not to waste them. You
are working in a public institution, where all you do and say,
and all that you yourselves *are,* has a wider influence for good
or evil than it would do in the narrower home circle, and we

cannot alter this fact by shutting our eyes to it. As nursing is so pre-eminently the woman's profession, what sort of women must you not resolve to be ?

If only all of you could understand, when you enter a hospital, that henceforth in a double sense you must "walk worthy of the vocation wherewith you are called," it would be very helpful to you, and it could scarcely fail to have a beneficial influence on your work. Let it make you the more careful, too, to remember that each one amongst you, individually, is more or less responsible for the credit of the whole institution. If any one of you behaves in such a way as to disgrace the uniform you wear, all the others suffer for it in the general estimation.

Each one of you who wins our certificate of training will have it in your power to make us proud of your connection with us in the future, or very sadly the reverse. You know how rejoiced men are when a member of their hospital or college has won distinction of any kind, and how they feel that his credit reflects itself to an extent upon them. Let it be the same with you. Many of you *can* be first-rate. It rests with you to make up your minds that you *will* be ; and having done so, how are you to set to work ?

I would have you consider a little some practical details concerning this much-talked-of hospital training, and such reflection will probably help you to banish a few of those preconceived notions concerning it which are apt to stand in the way of beginners. If you think of the subject as a whole, I believe you will share the opinion of those who have given much careful thought to the matter, and freely admit that it would be difficult to conceive any system more calculated to produce good results than the one adopted here. The fact that you have perfectly regular and uninterrupted courses of lectures on nursing, and that each one of you is enabled to attend them all, is not a small advantage. Then the division

of these lectures into three sets, not only gives each branch
of your work due consideration, but of necessity, on a subject
of limited extent like nursing, it involves the repetition by each
lecturer of a great deal that has been said before, combined
with the new matter set before you, and this repetition of
essential details can scarcely fail to impress them upon your
minds. In addition to these lectures you have an increasingly
good library on the subject that you are here to study, and
every facility is afforded for you to avail yourselves of it, so
that even without your practical work in the wards your
theoretical knowledge of nursing should be excellent. The
combination of this with the advantage of actual personal
experience in the wards, has not only the merit of being
invaluable in itself, but adds at the same time a double
interest to the theory of your art, and leaves little else to be
provided for the efficiency of your training. The success of
these means must rest in a great measure upon your application of them individually, and in cases where they fail to
produce a good result there must be either the want of
capacity to excel or a grave error in the method with which
you have set to work.

It seems to me that some of you expect to be taught
exactly as though you were children. In teaching a child we
should frequently pause to ascertain how much had been
understood ; we should keep more or less to one point until
it was learnt perfectly, and if no pains were taken we might
say that nothing else should be done until the lesson was
accomplished. Obviously that is not a system by which
hospital nursing could be taught, any more than it is a
subject which children could study ; and it is desirable that
you should each have a clear idea in your minds of the way
in which you are to acquire proficiency. Children frequently
have no desire to learn. Presumably not one of you would
be here unless you had made up your mind, for some reason

or other, that you wished to be trained. If I may apply a
very homely simile to the matter, perhaps I may make my
meaning clear to you. If a dish of knowledge is placed
before you, you, being grown-up women, and wishing for
this knowledge, must *help yourselves* to it, or go away without
any. If you were little children we should feel it a duty to
go round with a spoon and feed you, and in that case we
should provide food for that process. As it is, we cannot
force you to swallow it ; such a proceeding would neither be
polite nor practicable. It is not possible for us to do more
than prepare this knowledge for your use in as palatable
a form as we are able, and entreat each one of you to partake
of as much as you possibly can. I say this to you that you
may recognize the value of your opportunities at the beginning, in order to avail yourselves of them. We can do
everything short of *making you learn ; that* you must do *for
yourselves.* If you do not clearly understand what you are
told, make a point of asking questions about it until you do.
Perhaps it may not be convenient to do so immediately ; but
then keep a rough note-book, and make memoranda of the
things you want to know, until a good opportunity offers of
getting them explained. Nothing would give me greater
pleasure than to attempt to solve some of your individual
difficulties for you ; but before I can do this, you yourselves must take the trouble to tell me what they are. Ask
the sisters or your fellow-workers, or any one you like, but
find out somehow, and persevere until you know. Do not
rest satisfied with having asked, remember, until you are
confident that you understand the matter so well that you
could explain it to another. It is not in the least discredit-
able to you to display ignorance on the most commonplace
detail of nursing *now.* You are not *expected* to know anything about it to begin with, even if it happens that you do.
If you knew all about hospital nursing it is not to be supposed

that you would devote at least two years of your life, as the majority of you intend, to the study of it; so do not let any fear of being laughed at for not knowing keep you from asking questions, and do not be discouraged from asking again in other directions if your attempts to find out what you wish to know have been unsuccessful. It is no disgrace to be ignorant *now*, but you will not be able to say the same at the end of your training, if you have failed to acquire what it was your duty to learn. If when it is your turn to teach— and remember every certificated nurse becomes an authority on the subject, at least to those who know nothing of it—if when you are asked the simple questions that you have a *right* to be asking yourselves now, you cannot give information to others because you have been too careless, too apathetic, or too silly to ask for it, I think *then* you might well be ashamed to confess that " you do not know."

If I have made myself clear to you, I can only beg you all to make up your minds to set about learning in the right way, and realize to what an important extent the quality of your training depends *upon yourselves.* We will not fail to do our part, and I want you to begin by doing your very best, applying your brightest energies to the task you have undertaken, with plenty of hope and courage to start with, and a good supply of steady perseverance to carry you through.

It is your first object to do your own duty faithfully and well, but do not forget that you must also help your fellow-workers to the utmost of your power. I have often heard both sisters and nurses exclaim, "I never shall forget my first day in a hospital!" Yet I am sometimes tempted to think they must forget very completely or be sadly deficient in sympathy, when they can fail to give a thoroughly cordial, friendly greeting to every new beginner with whom they come in contact. As I am addressing probationers chiefly, the recollection of your first appearance must still be fresh in your minds, and I hope for the sake of others that you will keep it so to some purpose. If you have been fortunate enough to be received in a kindly spirit by those with whom your practical work commenced, show a grateful remembrance of it by extending the right hand of fellowship *immediately* to every new-comer. Should they prove unworthy, it is time enough to withdraw it again, but give them some encouragement to start with. On the other hand, if you have little to be grateful for in this way, let the thought of the discomfort you experienced make you doubly eager to save others from it. I lay a good deal of stress on this commonplace incident, because it is one of those in which you can do so much to help each other, and in which I can do scarcely anything to help you. It may be that my sympathy with those going through the little ordeal of a first beginning is the more active because it occasionally happens that I know something of such circumstances as may have led them to take to this work. But be this as it may, however kindly disposed I may feel towards any stranger, *you* know that week after week may go by without much opportunity of my giving any evidence of it beyond the ordinary formal greeting. Whereas *you* are workers together, and may be of much service to each other. Another reason why I am careful to speak of this is that many of you may fail to overcome the shy awkwardness which some experience in speaking to a stranger, because they do not realize how thoroughly the effort is worth while. It is one of the little things apt to be left undone by the most good-natured simply from want of thought. Possibly there is a little tendency in a continuance of hospital life to produce the spirit which inquires, " Am I my brother's keeper ? " Guard against it, please.

Now, in order to become the sort of nurse that I have described to you there are various essential qualifications in which you can do much towards training yourselves, and without which nothing we can do for you will ever make you worthy of the name of a " trained nurse."

Truthfulness, obedience, and punctuality are simply indispensable qualities. Do guard yourselves against the many temptations which a nurse finds not to be strictly accurate. Forgetfulness is a fault for which a nurse should never excuse herself, but do own to that steadily rather than give a false impression. No one will lose confidence in you if you own your fault; they will see that you care more for what is right and for your patients than you do for yourself. It is degrading to your own character to be untrue, and it may be harmful in its result to your patients also. You will have to learn a great deal before it will be possible for you to give a thoroughly accurate report of your case, because to do this you will need to know more fully how and what to observe; but the very newest and most inexperienced among you can realize the importance of being extremely exact in your statements.

Prompt, intelligent, and careful obedience is perhaps of all others the distinguishing quality of a perfect nurse. It is the one which inspires the doctor with more trust in her than anything else will do, and which shows that she really understands her work. No one who has not acquired the habit of quiet obedience to orders, whether she happens to approve of them or not, has any right to be considered a " trained nurse." Implicit obedience is the clear duty of a probationer, and you must not add to the difficulties of those whose duty it is to rule by questioning what they say. The responsibility does not rest with you. There may be many excuses for ignorance on the part of the probationer, but be sure there can be none for disobedience.

And, while I am speaking on this subject, let me remind you of the duty you have to perform in the way of being very loyal to those under whom you are placed.

I know it is pleasant when you are able to love and admire those for whom and with whom you are working. It makes your work much brighter and easier, and I am always glad when you are fortunate enough to be able to do this. But when you have not the help of personal affection; when you feel that perhaps they are not treating you quite fairly, or are not setting you a good example in this respect by loyalty towards those in authority over them;—I want you to understand that no failure of duty on their part alters your duty towards them. You are not responsible for their faults, but you are for your own actions. It *is* a fault to speak against the head of a ward to those who have to work under her; so, whether you may happen to be right or wrong in your opinion, if you cannot sincerely praise, try and be silent. You can learn something from every one with whom you come in contact. It may be an example of what you would do well to copy, or it may be what you must take pains to avoid. In any case, it is not your part to criticize, though your judgment may be correct. Remember, you cannot quite judge of their difficulties until you have been in their place.

The regularity of hospital life is, or should be, helpful to you in gaining the habit of punctuality; and you must not be satisfied with yourselves, any more than I shall ever be satisfied with you, until you have become perfect in this respect. Why should you not be so? It only means taking a little trouble.

An unpunctual nurse has lost her patient before now by neglecting to administer the prescribed medicine or stimulants at *the right time*. It seems almost ridiculous that I should remind you that when food, medicine, applications, etc., are ordered at any particular time, it means that the patient is to have them at that hour, *not that you are to begin to get them ready*. But I have seen and known so many nurses fall into this error that I think it is necessary for me to point it out to you. Sometimes the consequences of these delays are serious, sometimes they are not important to the patient; but they are always important as indicating a slovenly habit in yourselves. If a poultice is ordered at a certain hour, try and have it ready when the clock strikes; do not wait for it to strike before you begin to think about making the poultice, and then rest under the delusion that you are punctual!

Do you see how much is required to make your work really trustworthy? I need not linger to speak of other nursing qualities, such as memory, forethought, cleanliness, calmness, cheerfulness, neatness. You know, without my telling you, how valuable they are, and what a difference all these things make.

The cultivation of what may be termed good hospital manners is another point to which I must call your attention. Not that I wish to make this of *equal* importance with the other things of which we have just been speaking, but because they must not be overlooked; and I think a few hints on the subject will be of service to you.

You can see for yourselves that manners which would be quite suitable at an entertainment, for instance, would not be adapted to a church, or behaviour that would be quite pleasant and comfortable in your own homes would not be at all proper in the streets. Hospitals are public buildings, and you must endeavour to remember this, and conduct yourselves accordingly. "Manners are not idle;" they indicate a great deal. Besides, they are much within our own control. It seems more natural to some than to others to have what we call " good manners; " but they can be acquired by every one with so little care and trouble, that there is no excuse for neglecting them.

A kindly, pleasant manner to your patients is of great importance. It is such a good quality for a nurse if it can truly be said of her that she never renders the most disagreeable service ungraciously; and you will add immensely to the gratitude, as well as to the comfort, of your patients if you try and act up to this. It will be well for yourselves, and for those with whom you come in contact, if you can always recollect that "if a thing has to be done at all, do it pleasantly."

Is it not curious that hospital nurses, beyond other people, should often completely forget the injunction, "Be pitiful, be courteous"? It is especially when your patients are weak and helpless and irritable that you need to be gentle and considerate towards them; they are so completely in your power, and they may so easily be made to suffer more than they need do, by your having a sharp way of speaking, a rough touch, or a grumbling manner of attending to them. You are giving up a part of your life to wait upon them; then surely it is worth while to do it cheerfully.

If you fail in these little ways, it *does* prove that you are lacking in true womanly pity and tenderness, and that you are so far unfitted for your post. The best guide for you to ascertain for yourselves whether you are failing or succeeding in this particular, is simply to judge, not whether you are more or less gentle than some of your fellow-workers, but whether you would like to have such offices as you may have to perform for your patients rendered in the same manner that you are adopting towards them. Remember that you can be perfectly kind to your patients, and yet never allow them to speak to you too familiarly or be on too free and easy terms with you.

Loud voices, and noisy, squeaking boots are thoroughly unnurselike, and often so distressing to patients, that I should scarcely have thought it necessary to speak of them, if I did not know, from daily experience, how slow some of you are to discover the importance of these very obvious defects. I am sure it cannot have occurred to some, who appear to think

it hard or unreasonable that they should be expected to
conform to the requirements of hospital life in such details,
what selfishness they display in allowing patients (who are
not exactly in a position to complain) to suffer discomfort—
to use no stronger word—rather than incur a certain amount
of inconvenience themselves ! I venture to think that women
who are not above such small considerations of personal
vanity are scarcely worthy to take up the work upon which
they have entered. Much character is displayed in little
actions of this kind, and selfishness is pre-eminently a defect
which disqualifies a woman for the nursing profession. It is
an evidence of such thoughtlessness that I do not wonder
doctors speak as they do of those who indulge in them. You
can easily understand for yourselves how objectionable these
disturbances are; and I wonder occasionally, when I see a
nurse rushing and clattering about, when perhaps the doctors
are using their stethoscopes, how it is they do not complain
of it even more ; but they can scarcely fail to notice the want
of perception which any one doing such a thing displays.

As far as your manner to the matron is concerned, I need
not say much, for I could not wish for anything pleasanter
than the consideration and the bright, ready courtesy I receive
from you all. But one point I will mention for your own
satisfaction, because the sisters have told me that you are
sometimes puzzled about it. When I am in the wards, unless
the sister is free to attend to me, I like whoever is doing staff-
nurse's duty, or, if she is in attendance on the medical
officers, any probationer that may be on duty there, to go
round with me. I like this for two reasons. One is that it
is convenient to have some one close at hand to answer any
question I may want to ask ; but the other, and perhaps the
stronger, reason is that this is one of the few opportunities
I have of speaking to you individually. We live such busy
lives that it is comparatively seldom that we come into personal

contact, and it is always a pleasure to me to meet those in whose welfare I feel so much interest. I am naturally reluctant to miss such opportunities as occur. I equally like you to accompany visitors when they are being taken round the ward, whether I am with them or any of the other hospital officials. Sometimes it may happen that you are helpful in answering questions. At any rate, it is always pleasant and desirable to see you at hand, so do not be afraid that you are in the way. Never remain seated when visitors are passing through your ward.

I must also remind you of the courtesy that is due from every member of the nursing staff to strangers who enter the wards unattended. It is an extremely awkward feeling to go into a ward, whatever your mission there may be, and find yourself completely ignored. If any of you have ever tried the experiment yourselves by going, as a stray visitor, to any other hospital, and should happen to have been greeted with the indifference of which I speak, I am confident that you will retain such a melancholy recollection of the event that you will never leave others to experience a similar fate. It is the distinct duty of the nurse in charge of the ward, or, if she is engaged at the moment, for any probationer present, to go up to any stranger who is hesitating where to go or what to do next, with the simple question, "Is there anything I can do for you?" The visitor may be of no special consequence, but your manners are always of importance; and it would distress me personally, and be a reflection upon all our nursing staff, if any member of it is found wanting in that ready courtesy and kindness which is admirable under all circumstances, and almost a necessity for those who are in any way connected with the public life of a hospital. I have heard that there are persons who, by some extraordinary perversion of ideas, are under the impresssion that it is derogatory to their dignity—or " beneath them," as I believe the phrase goes—to pay attention to such little matters as these, or to show the consideration, if I may venture to use the term, due from all wearing our hospital uniform to those who may address them, apart from any question of the social standing on either side. There are other persons, again—and I believe these are more numerous—who rather pride themselves on a certain abrupt curtness of speech, most unpleasant to those who have to submit to it, but which the speakers erroneously think amply atoned for by the explanation that it is " only my manner ! " If that is the case, the sooner it is altered the better it will be for all concerned. I refer to these delusions, though I hope no one here is labouring under them. It can do us no harm to be duly impressed with the practical truth conveyed in the poetical statement, that " the gentler born the maiden, . . . the more bound to be sweet and serviceable."

Next, with regard to your official manner to the sisters. Do not sit down, nor remain sitting, when the sister is giving you orders about the patients or your work. It is not polite, and does not look well. Of course, it is different if you are only talking together. The social position of yourselves or of the sister does not affect the question at all. This is simply the courtesy due to the sister of the ward from those working under her. She has too much to do to be constantly reminding you ; but be particular about these little things for your own sakes ; it may be that you will want to teach them to others by-and-by.

Probationers and nurses must not report anything to the medical officers in the presence of the sister. If there is any information that should be made known, the probationer must tell the sister, and it is for her to report it to the medical officer. Sisters are responsible for all that goes on in their ward, and it is your duty to help them, by keeping them promptly and carefully informed of any points con-

nected with the patients; but you must avoid taking her
place when she is there. If you are attending to the medical
officer without the sister, then, of course, you must give him
all the necessary information; but it is a very "untrained"
thing for a nurse or probationer to answer or ask questions,
or give reports, when the sister is in attendance.

I am very distinct and definite about these small things,
because, when you are once told, you need not forget them;
and I am confident that many of you will feel helped by
knowing what is correct in these little matters. It is not
possible to know them by instinct, and it is a disagreeable
experience to find them out by making mistakes. Of course,
you will never think of sitting down or of remaining seated
while you are speaking or being spoken to by *any* of the
medical staff, whether a senior or junior member of it,
including the dressers and students; it looks unbusiness-like
and unprofessional. There is, again, no question of social
equality or inequality involved in this; but if you forget it,
those who are capable of judging will know at once that you
are ignorant of ordinary details of hospital routine. You
cannot always help other people's manner to you, but you can
do a great deal towards making it what you wish to have it,
and at any rate you can always help yours to them. It is
not by being frivolous and silly, nor solemn and disagreeable,
that you will hold your own and keep others in their place,
but by a quiet, pleasant, gentle manner to *all* those with
whom you come in contact.

Think of the harm you do if you give one man cause to
think and speak worse of women than before he entered the
hospital. Give your fellow-workers a chance of respecting
as well as of liking you, and they will not fail to do so.
Remember that it depends upon *you*, not upon them, whether
they are to leave the hospital declaring that they would not
have their sisters take up such a life for the world, or

whether you will have unobtrusively shown them a little bit
of what is meant by the "beauty of holiness"—as perhaps
only a good woman can do—and have taught them that a
hospital nurse is not the sort of person to be lightly spoken
of or idly trifled with, but one whose interest is centred in
quite other things. You must not leave it for others to help
you to do this. Why should they take the trouble? But
no one can hinder you, neither will they try to do so, if they
see that you are sincere and in earnest. All affectation is
contemptible and patent to all observers.

If these little details of manner do not strike any new
probationer joining you—and it is quite likely they will not—
take an early opportunity of giving her a quiet hint on the
subject, because it will prevent her looking awkward and
feeling uncomfortable on another occasion.

Be careful not to get into a habit of leaning up against
the tables and chairs, and the patients' beds, under any circumstances. It always gives an impression of slovenliness,
and, moreover, is quite unnecessary. On the other hand,
take every legitimate opportunity of sitting down and of
resting your feet, for you all have a great deal of standing;
and the more you can save yourselves in this way, the better
it is for you. If you could remember to put your feet up,
instead of only sitting down, when you are off duty, and not
walking, you would be much more refreshed and rested. Most
nurses suffer a great deal with their feet when they first
begin hospital work, and it often makes them feel very tired
when they are quite well otherwise.

It is part of a sensible woman's duty to take proper care
of her own health; because, however good your intentions
may be, you cannot do your work, nor yourself justice, *for
long*, when you are not well. Plenty of fresh air, and as
much change of scene as possible, are most necessary for
you; and the patients, too, get the benefit of it, by your

being all the brighter on your return to them. Try and
resist the inclination to stay in because you are tired; you
will nearly always be glad afterwards, if you have summoned
up sufficient energy to go out. Hospital work is very absorbing, and it is not at all good for you to get your views of life
narrowed by taking no interest in other things. Nurses, of
all people, ought to understand that it is impossible to
keep well and in good working order without regular meals
and fresh air, and both are specially important to those who
are on night duty.

One other little thing I must just remind you of, while
I am speaking about yourselves, and that is the extreme
care you must always remember to take in covering up any
scratch or cut you may have on your hands, if it is ever so
small, while you are in the wards of a hospital. It is not
being fussy to do this, but it simply shows that you have
sufficient common sense not to risk poisoning your hand. It
is some little trouble, but nurses *must* take care of their
hands. If you have forgotten to cover any little place where
the skin has broken, before doing a dressing, immediately
wash it in carbolic, and remedy the omission without further
delay. Nurses *ought* not to get bad fingers, but they inevitably will do so unless they take every precaution. Carbolic
hardens the hands very much, as most of you know, but you
can keep them soft with glycerine; and if you are going to
put them into anything very disagreeable, you can fill your
nails with soap. It is much pleasanter for your patients to
be touched by you if you keep your hands and nails in as
nice condition as you can, and it is an important habit for
yourself. I was asked the other day if I could do anything
to assist a nurse who had been obliged to have her right arm
amputated, from having poisoned her finger with a case she
was nursing. I tell you this, not to make you nervous, but
to convince you that you cannot be careless in this respect
without grave risk to yourselves.

Now, there are one or two faults and temptations which people living together in a public institution somewhat readily fall into, and against which it is well for you to be on your guard. I dare say many of you will agree with me at once when I mention the two most prevalent as being gossip and grumbling.

A hospital is a little world in itself, and I fear the small-minded notions, spite, and jealousy which too often prevail, make the conversation of a household of women almost proverbial in this most undesirable way. If it were possible to put together the time which is spent in any one building of this kind in one day, in these two most unprofitable occupations, how many hours would have been thus wasted?

Gossip *may* do an immense amount of harm; it *can* do no possible good. The idle stories of each other, or of those with whom you are working, merely repeated and listened to for amusement, are often not entirely true; and, if they do not fail in this respect, they are not quite kind, and you feel hurt and annoyed yourselves when you find that others have been doing the same about you. It is not enough "not to *mean* any harm; you must not *do* any. Each one of you can do a great deal by making a personal effort not to indulge in the general tendency to gossip, and by distinctly showing that you take no interest in such things when others begin to speak of them.

Grumbling is a little different from gossip, inasmuch as it does the person who grumbles more harm than anybody else, though the harm done by no means ends there. When you have a discontented patient in the wards, who will not be pleased with anything you do, no matter what trouble you take, have you not noticed how soon the dissatisfied spirit spreads, and how inclined to complain nearly all the others become? I need scarcely point out to you that it is the same in every other community.

I do not think we have any right to make life harder for others. I am sure you each find difficulties to overcome, without having them increased by any thoroughly depressing companions. I consider that it is simply due to our best workers that those whose influence has no tendency for good in this respect should, as far as possible, be excluded from our number. I am far from saying that you never have anything to grumble at, but I do emphatically say that, whatever your grievance may be, grumbling is not the way to mend it. Do not misunderstand me and think that I wish you to put up with everything you do not like, without mentioning it. I mean, speak of it only to those who have the power to alter it. That would be complaining to some purpose, and is a very different thing from idly spreading a feeling of discontent that helps nobody.

Try and remember as much as you can, when you find things irksome to you, that those in authority *are* sincerely desirous of doing what is best for all; and if you cannot always see this, and do not agree with their view of the matter, whatever it may be, at least this conviction will render it less difficult for you to do your part.

If you can keep from gossiping and grumbling, you will be all the happier yourselves, and a helpful example to your fellow-workers. I am sure, if you pause to think of it, you will agree with me, that, "It is better to fight for the good than to rail at the ill." Success in guarding against or in conquering these two deplorable failings will be well worth the constant effort involved in gaining it. Nurses get into these habits before they are aware of it themselves, just because "everybody does it;" but if you will resolve individually to fight against them, I am confident that we shall have reason to be satisfied with the result.

I cannot resist quoting to you a remark of Sir Frederick Leighton's that I came across the other day. "Believe me,"

he says, " whatever of dignity, whatever of strength we have
within us, will dignify and make strong the labours of our
hands; whatever littleness degrades our spirit, will lessen
them and drag them down.   Whatever noble fire is in our
hearts will burn also in our work; whatever purity is ours
will chasten and exalt it; for as we are, so our work is; and
what we sow in our lives, that beyond a doubt we shall reap,
for good or for ill, in the strengthening or defacing of whatever gifts have fallen to our lot."

Those words appear to me to be full of encouragement.

I shall endeavour in our next lectures to give you some
definite instruction on the different practical details of nursing,
but it seemed essential that we should get a clear idea of the
type of woman that a nurse herself should be, before we
could reasonably begin to talk about the various items of
her work.   I earnestly hope that what I have said may be of
service and have weight with you, and that each one of you
will deliberately resolve to attain, as nearly as possible, to
the high standard of nurses and nursing which I have tried
to set before you.

> " Greatly begin; if you have time
> But for one line—be that sublime:
> Not failure, but low aim is crime."

LECTURE II.

In our last lecture we dwelt chiefly upon two important questions, namely, what trained nursing is, and the personal qualifications desirable for a nurse. We also considered to some extent the distinction between the work of doctors and nurses, and the relation they bear to each other in their work. We spoke of the similarity in the object of each, as far as the cure and relief of the sick and suffering are concerned, and of the difference that it is essential for each to observe and maintain for the efficient attainment of that object.

I need scarcely take up your time with the repetition in detail of what these distinctions are. I will only briefly remind you that the diagnosis of the case and the laying down of a scientific plan of treatment is the work of the doctor. It is as an active agent in carrying out that plan of treatment that the important work of the nurse lies. The doctor prescribes; for the most part it is left to you to carry out that prescription, and it is obvious that the welfare of the patient must depend upon the efficiency and mutual help of doctor and nurse. Any misapprehension of the relationship you bear to each other, any aggressive tendencies on the part of the nurse, and any want of confidence on the part of the doctor can but have a disadvantageous effect upon work which probably you are both desirous of making as perfect as possible. Doctors can often do so little without nurses that they are frequently the first to acknowledge that " nearly everything depends upon the nursing." This is a familiar phrase to us in reference to many cases. On the other hand, it is only right in deference to the far longer, wider, and to a great extent different range of studies of doctors, that nurses should help them to carry out whatever means they may think fit to adopt by prompt and intelligent obedience.

It follows, therefore, that nurses have to turn their attention to the best means of carrying out whatever details may be considered under the head of " treatment."

We shall find it helpful to recognize the fact that treatment usually presents itself to us under one or more of three aspects. First, it may be necessary to provide an antidote to any poison and to remove all sources of harm; secondly, the chief consideration may be to place and to keep the patient in the most favourable condition for self-cure; thirdly, it may be desirable to aid in treatment by drugs which experience or experiment have shown to be efficacious.*

Sometimes only one method of treatment may be employed, sometimes two, and frequently all three are brought into requisition; but you will find that almost every case of which you can think will come under one or more of these heads, and we will, therefore, make them the plan for the first part of this course of lectures. I shall probably make my meaning more clear to you by one or two illustrations.

Let us suppose a case of typhoid fever to be due to the defective drainage or water of the locality in which the

* Amongst much other valuable help I am particularly and entirely indebted to Dr. Allchin for this system of arranging the subject. I am aware that I have not extended this classification to the fullest possible limit which it is capable of being extended to, and which those who have the privilege of being acquainted with Dr. Allchin's own lectures cannot fail to appreciate. I am none the less under much obligation to him for a method which has enabled me to regard the whole nursing question from a clear point of view, and which I trust may be of equal service in teaching others to look at it in a plain, practical light.

patient is living. Directly the doctor had ascertained this, he would insist upon the removal of the patient to some place free from these pernicious influences, and thus, in the first place, he would carry out the treatment which I have spoken of under the first heading, and "remove all sources of harm." But he would not stop there, and consider that all the treatment necessary for a patient suffering from typhoid fever was to place him in healthy surroundings, though he might reasonably believe all other means useless without this essential preliminary.

Without entering into all the details of nursing typhoid fever, most of you know that all solid food is carefully with-held, that the patient is not allowed to sit up, much less to stand or walk about. You do not *cure* typhoid fever by carrying out the usual instructions on these points, but by taking these precautions you give the disease from which the patient is suffering, the best chance of running a favourable course, and thus carry out the treatment spoken of under the second heading, *i.e.*, "placing the patient in the most favour-able condition for self-cure."

But the doctor will probably consider it desirable to aid in treatment by drugs which experience or experiment have shown to be efficacious; and thus all three methods would be combined for the successful treatment of one case.

On the other hand, one form of treatment may be sufficient. Supposing a person to have swallowed a poison, it may be possible to administer the direct antidote [to it, as strong coffee after opium poisoning, or any alkali if an acid poison has been taken, or if a patient working in a lead-factory begins to show symptoms of lead-poisoning, he may regain health and strength by changing his occupation, and so "remove all sources of harm;" thus the treatment spoken of under the first heading would prove sufficient. Then, if a man has broken his leg, the only thing you can do is to put him

and it in the most favourable position for self-cure, by procuring the necessary rest and position, so that Nature may
perform her own cure without interruption. In this case the
treatment spoken of under the second heading is all that would
be required. Again, there are circumstances in which different
drugs may be considered likely to produce a beneficial effect
upon the system without other remedies being necessary, so
that the treatment spoken of under the third heading is occasionally employed alone, but this is more often used in combination with one or both of the other forms of treatment.
Now, to repeat the statement with which I started, for the
sake of clearness, you will remember that treatment nearly
always presents itself under one or more of three aspects.
First, to provide an antidote to any poison, and to remove
all sources of harm; secondly, to put the patient under the
most favourable condition for self-cure : thirdly, to aid in
treatment by drugs which experience or experiment have
shown to be efficacious.

In order to make this fact your own, just think of the
various cases in your respective wards, and settle in your own
minds for your own satisfaction—not necessarily for anybody
else's benefit or information, remember—under which of these
headings the treatment of your different patients comes, for
each case could be placed under one or more of them.

Treatment consists in the application of natural agents,
such as rest, heat, cold, light, electricity, etc., adapted to the
special needs of each particular case. Some of you will already
have thought for yourselves that it is under the second
heading that most of a nurse's work comes. To place and
to keep the patient in the most favourable condition for self-
cure usually involves more nursing than it appears to do at
first sight.

" Rest " is the natural agent that is constantly employed in
various degrees as a means of treatment. Rest may be

complete or comparative, and it may be applied to the entire
body, as by absolute rest in bed, or locally, as applied to
different parts of the body by means of splints, bandages, or
other mechanical arrangements. A nurse's duty in carrying
out the treatment of absolute rest in bed includes bed-making
for general and for helpless cases, with the washing and other
attentions needed for such patients as are unable or forbidden
to help themselves. So I propose to deal first with the details
involved in the nursing of a case where the order of complete
rest in bed has been given. The feeding of helpless patients
we will speak of when we consider the administration of
food; but I think we may finish all that needs to be said on
these other points to-night.

First, with regard to bedsteads.

The superiority of iron or brass over every species of
wooden bedsteads is so universally acknowledged that I need
not do more than allude to the fact.

For nursing the sick it is essential that bedsteads should
not be too wide. This is an important consideration, and one
that is frequently overlooked in private nursing. It is impossible to move the patient, to change the sheets, or to
attend to a helpless case with any degree of comfort if the
bed is too wide. If there is an idea of affording the patient
relief by changing him from side to side, this plan can be
executed infinitely better by means of two smaller beds that
can be put next each other, for the purpose of lifting the
patient to a fresh place; and the bed which he has just
vacated can then be moved away without disturbing him,
and the nurse remains able to get at her patient in all
directions in a manner that will contribute greatly to his
comfort. In hospitals, of course, these matters do not rest
with you; but many of you are training for private nursing,
and it is well to have studied them. For patients who are
able to get in and out of bed, it will fatigue them less if the

bedstead is no higher than a sofa; but for bedridden cases rather a high bedstead is less tiring for the nurse, and does not affect the comfort of the patient in any way. Bedsteads should never be placed with one side against a wall, except for the purpose of keeping a delirious patient in bed, for such an arrangement materially adds to the difficulty of attending to the patient's wants. Nothing can be cleaner or nicer than the chain spring bedstead. That, with a hair mattress, is the best arrangement I know out of many good ones for all ordinary cases.

Sometimes water beds are ordered, and they are extremely useful in some cases where pressure must be specially avoided. When you have to prepare them, remember they must not be too full, nor quite cold. If you find it most convenient to nearly fill them with cold water, add a few jugs of hot water to conclude with, that there may be no feeling of chill when the patient is placed on it. The same rule applies to the filling of water pillows. As a rule, these beds are not very popular; the patients frequently complain of a feeling of "sea-sickness."

A spring bed, with a hair mattress and a square water pillow, is generally the most conducive to comfort if the choice happens to rest with you; but if the doctor for whom you are nursing prefers otherwise, that settles the question of course. I should say that, as a rule, circular water pillows are preferred in theory, and square water pillows in practice; but there, again, circumstances must decide, and many may differ from this opinion.

Beds for cases of fracture and others for special cases we can consider when we come to the nursing of those cases; they must be made hard with boards or straw mattresses, unless the bedsteads are made for special cases, such as our fracture femur bedsteads here. Flock beds are distressing to a nurse's, as well as to a patient's, feelings. They are so difficult to get into shape, to keep free from lumps, and to make comfortable. The sole merit they possess for hospital use is cleanliness. They can be easily replenished; but I can only hope that we shall shortly have the satisfaction of seeing them all replaced by spring bedsteads and hair mattresses. I do not think that with the shape of iron bedstead now in use any theory on the subject of ventilation being impeded by curtains deserves sufficient importance to be seriously considered, as opposed to the great advantage of the comparative privacy they afford, particularly in large wards like ours, where the publicity is unavoidably extreme. It is a great comfort to many, not only to be able to put themselves partially out of sight, but to be able to shut out some of the distressing sights which occasionally surround them. Provided curtains are of a washing material, and changed often enough to ensure cleanliness, and that they are not arranged in any manner calculated to interfere with ventilation to any appreciable extent, my own opinion is strongly in favour of them, except, of course, for infectious cases. I am aware that many differ from my view of this question, and it is merely a matter of opinion whether the advantages or disadvantages of allowing curtains to be used exceed each other. I believe them to be a very desirable comfort in the charge of a careful nurse, [but I also admit that a careless nurse may allow them to become a source of positive danger, in every case where there is the slightest possibility of any kind of infection being harboured by them.

It does not rest with you at present to choose the position of beds for your patients; but any of you who are training with a view to employing your knowledge of nursing outside the walls of a hospital, will find that the choice of all this mainly depends upon you, and you will often be expected to understand and explain, not only *what* is best, but *why* it is best.

If the bed can be placed so that the patient can see out of window, so much the better. Let the light fall fully though crossways on the patient, if possible; the doctor always prefers it. You can shut out light when needful, but you can never make it come through a blank wall. Some people have an idea that it is orthodox to keep a sick room rather dark. With a few exceptions, it is best to brighten up your ward or sick room with as much sunshine as you can possibly get into it. Of course, you would not allow your patient to lie with the sunshine streaming into his eyes; but unobservant nurses are apt to forget that the sun does not remain in the same position all day, and that if it has been necessary to draw down the blind for a time, it may soon be desirable to pull it up again. A dark-green blind is best for keeping out the light. Sunshine is almost a necessity, and has a definite and powerful influence for good, physically as well as morally.

If your patient is well enough to be moved out of bed while it is made, take care that he is warmly wrapped up with a blanket, and that his bare feet are not left touching the floor. In some cases a foot-warmer is desirable; for the fact that the bed will be made in a very few minutes is no reason for letting your patient feel cold, or experience any other avoidable discomfort during the process.

Bed-making should be the first work of the day-nurse and probationer when they enter the ward in the morning. The sister must always be asked if the patient may be allowed to move out of bed while it is made, whenever there is the slightest doubt in the matter, for it is all important that some cases should not be allowed to put their feet to the ground. It requires two to make the bed properly when the patient is in it. It is easier to explain the best method of changing the sheets for a helpless patient, so that you may thoroughly understand it, by a practical illustration in the wards; and no doubt some of you have been taught it there.   This varies according to the case.

The great object to be borne in mind is saving the patient all unnecessary pain and fatigue.   Remove all the top bedclothes, except the sheet or one blanket, which must be retained as a covering.   If the patient can be with safety turned on his side, one person should hold him comfortably in that position, while the other rolls the under sheet, which is to be removed, close up to the patient, the whole length of the bed, and tucks the clean sheet in on that side, placing the remaining half of it rolled up close to the sheet that is about to be taken away.   The patient should then be gently turned over on the other side, and held in that position by the person standing there, while the other promptly draws the sheet off the bed, pulling out and smoothly tucking in the clean sheet on that side also.   It is of extreme importance to guard against wrinkles and crumbs in the bed, and it requires no little care and ingenuity to do this with complete success. The tiniest rucks in the bedclothes are indescribably uncomfortable, and, moreover, are productive of bed sores, when the skin is in a very sensitive condition.   Never shake sheets, blankets, or, indeed, anything *over* the patient's bed, but always *away from it*.

The clean top sheet must be placed over the patient before the one which has been retained as a covering has been withdrawn ; and, remember, there is no occasion to give the patient all sorts of suffocating sensations, by drawing sheet and blankets over his head until they are all accumulated, and you are ready to turn the clothes down at the top.   If the blankets are so long that they need doubling back, this should be done generally at the bottom of the bed, and not so that the additional weight and warmth of bedclothes should lie across the chest.   I mention these very small points, because they are constantly neglected from sheer want of thought.

Next we come to the arrangement of the pillows, for which no absolute rule can be given, though every one knows that a patient's comfort in bed largely depends upon their skilful adjustment. The principle to keep in view is that pillows are intended to support the patient in the position that he wishes or is able to adopt. The lower part of the back always needs supporting; the shoulders must have room to lean back, and the top pillow must be placed in such a way as to support the head, without either tilting it forward or obliging it to fall back. The arrangement of pillows and cushions is a very individual matter; and, with these general principles for guidance, only observation and experience can teach you what is likely to suit each particular case. Nursing is supposed by some to consist mainly in that graceful task known as "smoothing the pillow;" but, though we may smile at the familiar expression, we must not forget that it is distinctly refreshing to have the pillows shaken up occasionally, and the cool side placed next the patient. But one word of warning in reference to shaking up pillows. Never shake your pillows *on the bed*. It is wholly unnecessary to shake up your patient at the same time; and though in many cases jerks would not be disturbing, they are always carefully to be avoided. I dare say it strikes you that your own common sense would teach you this; but notice the first time that you are tempted to do it, or that you see some one else do it, and you will find that my warning is not superfluous, and that the next instance will occur sooner than you anticipate.

Draw-sheets and mackintoshes are managed in exactly the same way as the under sheet, but of course those can be changed in less time.

Some cases are best moved in a similar manner to that which I have just described, from the top to the bottom of the bed, instead of lengthways; but these are the exception, the other is the rule.

D

In some German hospitals tapes are sewn on to the mackintoshes and draw-sheets, and they are tied to the sides of the bed. It is a good plan, as it keeps them in place and free from wrinkles, but it involves a great deal of trouble. I do not know any English hospital in which it is done. Every accident bed should be made up with a mackintosh and draw sheet. Do not wait for the mattress to be saturated before discovering that one is necessary. Never put a blanket on the mattress under the patient, unless specially ordered to do so ; " it retains damp, and acts like a poultice," * and is, consequently, likely to induce bed sores. When patients are ordered to lie between blankets, place one *over* the bottom sheet, and put the top sheet over the blankets and next the counterpane or check, so that the bed may look neat.

The top sheet should not be tucked in at the bottom of the bed, but folded neatly back—over the blankets in those cases where the bedclothes will have to be turned back in that way for the surgeon, and back upon itself in those cases where the blankets can be tucked in at the bottom of the bed. It not only looks neater, but leaves the end smooth to put over the bolster when you use it for the under sheet and put a clean one on the top later on.

When you are going to make the bed, always place a chair or something to throw the clothes over, and never under any circumstances throw them on the floor, where, of course, they will catch up dust and dirt. I should scarcely have thought it necessary to tell you this, but I have so frequently seen them left on the ground.

You must not let the sides or the ends of blankets be seen dangling below the check or counterpane. It looks extremely untidy, and, moreover, they get dirty. Turn

---

* Miss Florence Nightingale's " Notes on Nursing." Amongst others, the short chapter on " Beds and Bedding " may be studied with advantage to all interested in this subject.

back the corners over the pillows crossways if they are
too long.

Hospital bedsteads should never have foot-pieces, and I
hope the day will come when we shall see no more of them.
In surgical wards it is almost impossible to use them, they so
interfere with a convenient position for putting on splints,
dressings, and bandages. They are less objectionable in medical
wards; but even there it is more difficult to make the beds look
neat with them. In places where linen checks are used, as in
this hospital, they should be tidily pinned round the foot of
the bed to keep them straight and smooth. At hospitals where
thicker counterpanes are used they are folded in such a manner
as to produce the same result, but the lighter material is altogether preferable. It is generally considered that scarlet
blankets form the best sort of coverlets for the use of the sick.
It is popularly supposed that they help to keep away fleas, but
I will not vouch for the truth of this supposition! Scarlet
coverlets look bright in a ward, but the glare of the colour
may prove a little trying to some sick people. Notice, if
a patient is restless, whether his bedclothes are too heavy.
Sometimes that makes all the difference to a weak patient,
and it is one of the points for a good nurse to pay attention
to when she finds that a patient is tossing about and uncomfortable without knowing why.

Whilst speaking of bedclothes, I may as well remind you
that in uncovering a patient for the doctor, you must avoid
exposing him more than is necessary. For instance, when
the feet or legs are to be examined, turn back the bedclothes from the foot. In some operation cases, such as
lithotomy, etc., the bed is made in such a way as to facilitate
the removal of the bedclothes in the middle. For examination
of the chest or abdomen the clothes are, of course, turned
down from the top, or it is a good plan to fold back the
check and blankets, and leave the top sheet over the patient

as a light covering which the doctor can move at his convenience without making the patient uncomfortable. In obstetric cases it is generally best to fold the clothes back from the side of the bed.

There is no need to expose the patient in making or remaking the bed, a process that is so often necessary with those delirious patients who are possessed with an unceasing desire to get up. You can always leave a blanket over the patient while you put on the sheet and other things, and then slip it out and put it on properly afterwards.

I must not conclude this subject without a word on the importance of airing the bed and body linen of those under your care, not only before it is used, when the damp is at any rate comparatively clean, but when it has been saturated with moisture from the skin, which is far more unwholesome.

In hospitals you have not generally a very large supply of body linen for your patients, but if you are obliged to put on soiled things again, at least you can air them thoroughly, and make them as dry and wholesome as the circumstances will permit before replacing them.

You can scarcely realize, unless you have experienced it, the comfort, and, moreover, the actual benefit a patient will derive, from having a shirt or blanket which has grown moist, cold, and offensive with emanations from the skin, replaced with a dry, warm one.

Of course it does not rest with you, as probationers, at present to decide when these changes may be made, but keep the importance of them in your minds, and do not forget that when you remove a patient's shirt, for the purpose of washing him, for instance, that it had better be airing by the fire ready to put on warm and dry, than lying on the bed for you to replace it in the same condition as it was taken off. Those of you who are preparing for private nursing should remember that it is not well to allow any airing of clothes, clean or otherwise, in the patient's room. In some hospitals we are not quite able to help ourselves in this respect.

In the children's ward we change their bedgowns and jackets for the night and the day, because it is so much more wholesome, and whenever you have an opportunity of persuading any other patients to do the same, there can be no doubt it is best for them.

Washing hospital patients is generally rather a formidable undertaking, and in most cases prompt ablutions are quite indispensable. Of course injured limbs must be very gently handled, if they are able to be cleansed at all, and mackintoshes should be used to prevent the sheets getting damp.

The nurse of a ward should see that the feet of all the patients are washed at least once a week, and it may in almost all cases be done without running any risk for the patient, provided that they are properly dried, and not allowed to remain cold.

In the daily washing of those patients who are incapable of washing themselves, only uncover the part you are doing at one time, and do not keep them with chest and arms exposed while you are washing the face. Do not begin the process and then leave them with the water drying in, while you run off to fetch a towel. It is such an uncomfortable thing to be washed instead of being able to wash one's self, that you must try to make it as little disagreeable as you can.

Get everything you want before you begin, and then wash your patient quickly and gently, without leaving off in the middle if you can help it, and take care not to wet the sheet or nightdress here and there, so as to leave your patient damp and disturbed, instead of refreshed. It will be a distinct pleasure and refreshment to some patients to have their face and hands sponged occasionally if it is skilfully done, without any wearisome fuss of preparation for the process which is sometimes such an effort to those in a weak condition.

The habit of washing several patients in one water is so exceedingly dirty, that I should hardly have supposed any nurse would have dreamt of doing such a thing did I not know to the contrary. Children are victimized most in this way, partly, I suppose, because the number to wash makes it a serious piece of business in their wards, and partly because they cannot object to it, as adult patients would do. When you think how utterly distasteful it would be to *you* to use water in which another *healthy* person had previously washed, I hope you can conceive what it is for sick people suffering from various diseases to be cleansed—if we can call it so—in the same water. Such a proceeding is not without risk either, and it is inexcusable for laziness and the slovenly desire to save yourselves trouble in this respect, to prevent your taking proper care of those dependent upon you.

I have not said a word about the extreme importance of keeping your patients perfectly clean, literally from their heads to their feet, because I may take it for granted that from the time when you first saw in the hospital how dirty people *can* be, you would understand that it is a nurse's first duty to pay constant attention to this essential of her patient's health and comfort.

Now we come to another very important point in which patients kept wholly at rest in bed are dependent upon you. I mean the skilful placing and removal of bed-pans and other utensils, and the care necessary for their perfect cleanliness and immediate removal from the wards after use. I need scarcely point out to you that to keep the air of a sick room, and still more of a ward, as fresh as it should be, great attention must be paid to the *immediate* removal of all excretions and other offensive matters.

The use of any chamber utensil without a lid is quite inexcusable, and even with a lid it must under no circumstances be allowed to remain for a moment in the ward after the patient has finished with it. If you have any doubt in your minds as to the absolute necessity of this rule, look at the inside of the lid when it has been in use for a few minutes. You will find it covered with condensed offensive moisture, which, if the lid had not been there, must have passed into the air, perceptibly poisoning it. It is impossible to be too particular about this rule. It is very important for yourselves, as the chief risk of nurses taking the infection from some diseases lies in this direction. It is more considerate for the feelings of the patient on whom you are attending, and the others in the ward, and it is essential for the ventilation. In many cases it is best to have some disinfectant at the bottom of the utensil before it is used, and in almost all cases a little clean water should be put there. It absorbs smell, and enables you to clean the vessel with greater facility.

If ever the choice of lids rests with you, there can be no doubt that earthenware is the cleanest material. The disadvantages of them are that they are rather noisy, unless gently handled, and they are liable to breakage. But they are certainly best, because earthenware does not become saturated with matter as unglazed wood is apt to do. The lids should be kept as scrupulously clean as the utensils themselves, and no really good nurse will ever be unmindful of these details, or think them beneath her. Great care must always be taken to keep the urine bottles also in a condition of perfect cleanliness. It is only those who have not thoroughly understood the subject who think " it does not matter."

In well-managed and efficiently nursed wards no chambers, even when clean, should ever be kept under the patient's bed in the daytime. I never want you to sacrifice the patient's comfort, or the utility of any arrangement, merely for the sake of appearances; but, on the other hand, it is a pity to sacrifice appearances more than is absolutely necessary Besides, keeping unsightly articles about in the ward, even when they are in a sanitary condition, increases the risk that they may not be removed with the same promptitude when they have been used, as they would be if fetched at the time they were required.

I see no objection to the habit of placing clean chambers under each bed when the ward has been duly settled for the night. The best custom is for the day nurse or probationer to carry out this arrangement the last thing before leaving the wards. It is the work of the night nurse or probationer to remove them in the morning, when she attends to any special instructions given in reference to individual cases in respect to the saving or measurement of urine or fæces, and this rule prevents any difficulty or mistakes in getting a clear report left for the medical officer. It is the duty of the day and night staff of nurses to leave the utensils perfectly clean for each other. Under no circumstances, day nor night, should bed-pans or slipper bed-pans be allowed to remain in the wards. I earnestly hope you will all take great pains with yourselves about being absolutely trustworthy in these details. The necessary care involves constant trouble, but that must never deter a conscientious nurse from being scrupulously careful about these things.

The bed-pan should be warmed, in cases where the patient is very sensitive to chill, by placing a little warm water in it prior to using it. The nurse must remember to wipe the edges afterwards. The bed-pan should be oiled for those cases where there is much perspiration, as in rheumatic fever, for instance. So much real pain and discomfort can be spared to patients by a skilful nurse, painstaking in these respects.

For patients who are able to raise themselves a little, you

should take the utensil in your left hand, and put your right hand gently and firmly under the patient's back, with the palm next to the patient's skin. If the patients are weak, it will give a sensation of support, and with a little practice this alone will enable you to know whether the vessel is in its proper position. It *is* so hard upon the patients in their weakness to be left in a damp, uncomfortable condition through the ignorance or clumsy carelessness of the person who ought to be their greatest help. If patients cannot raise themselves in the least, always ask another person to help you in placing them on and taking them off the bed-pan, and do not attempt to push it in or drag it out by main force. In the delicate condition which the skin of such patients is certain to be in, that alone is sufficient to induce a bed sore. It is no proof of a nurse's skill to do badly herself what it takes two people to do well, and even private nurses can generally procure the slight assistance necessary for these occasions.

If a bed sore exists, and the dressings are soiled and have to be removed at the same time, remember that a nurse must take them up with her forceps, and burn them at once, *not* leave them to stop up pipes, as is often too carelessly done.

The constant keeping of your patients dry and clean is most important, for many reasons that I need scarcely pause to point out to *you*—who must already know something of the matter—whether they are in a condition to call your attention to their wants or not. This is one of the many disagreeable duties which fall to your share, and which for that reason demands the utmost delicacy and kindness from you. Some patients are so considerate that it is almost a pleasure to attend to them, and others so careless or oblivious of the trouble they give that it is difficult to be patient with them ; but you will remember that the cultivation of a nice habit in this respect is invaluable to yourself, and will help you to get

through your trying work creditably. There have been too
many nurses careless of the distress they may cause their
patients by keeping them waiting for the assistance of which
they are in need. The only comment I can make upon this
is the very obvious one that the woman who *could* do such a
thing knowingly must indeed have mistaken her vocation.

And, finally, we come to the mental rest which a true
nurse will afford to her patient, and a very important point
this is, though it is more difficult to define than the practical
duties.

You want to "think for" your patients, and not leave
them the responsibility, which they will feel, whether acknowledged or otherwise, of thinking for themselves. Do not
answer them impatiently, and tell them it is "your business"
if they venture to remind you of anything, as I am sorry to
say I have heard an impatient nurse do, but still try and
think for them so carefully that they shall feel a sort of
restful confidence in you. *That* in itself is a tangible help to
a very weak patient.

To this end you must strenuously cultivate a self-con-
trolled manner. It is no excuse for exciting your patients to
say that you were "all in a hurry," or that you "never gave
it a thought." A nurse who screams because she is a little
startled, who flies aimlessly about in all directions if she is
asked for two or three things at once, who says by way of
explaining why she lost her head in an emergency that she
was "all in confusion," has much to learn. Why should you
be "all in confusion" whatever happens? Is it not because
you do not know any better? It *does* require practice, but
self-control *must* be gained if you are to be thoroughly
efficient. Moreover, a want of self-control is selfish, as showing that you do not put your patient first. It is ignorant,
too, I am afraid; showing great want of "training." How
many of you will let me say by-and-by that you are calm,

quick, quiet, gentle nurses? *Now* you are at the beginning of your training, and I do not want to expect too much of you, but I fear that it has to be acknowledged of many nurses, new and more experienced, that they are often noisy, bustling, excitable, and very easily flurried.

Unless you have been very ill yourself, you have no notion how weak patients depend for their own courage on their nurse's strength, and a quiet, confident manner will be an immense help to them. Even if you feel excited, or confused and worried, try hard not to *show* it.

You must cease to look upon this failing as excusable, but remember it is a grave defect in itself, and if you do not acquire this calm manner by the end of your training, you will never be first-rate. How I should like all nurses to become illustrations of a beautiful description I once read, though at this moment I cannot recall by whom it was written—

> " A calm, hushed presence
> Bringing rest—to those who felt and understood
> The dignity of womanhood."

In providing perfect rest, remember that much depends, too, upon night nurses. I cannot reprehend too strongly the deplorable custom that was once so prevalent in the hospital world, and which, I fear, is by no means extinct even yet, of putting the least efficient and the least dependable nurses on night duty. It is not too much to say that it was a common practice to put persons who were acknowledged to be totally unfit for day duty, in charge of wards at night, when, as all of you know, the responsibility which rests in their hands is at least double that which, in the ordinary course of things, can devolve upon any staff nurse on day duty. I have no doubt that this plan originated partly in the difficulty of finding night nurses, partly because culpable neglect of duty was more likely to remain undiscovered in

most cases by night than by day, and therefore gave less
trouble; but we can scarcely realize too strongly how wrong
and unjustifiable such a system is. This is scarcely the
occasion for me to enter into the many reasons why I dis-
approve of allotting the work of day and of night nursing to
an entirely distinct and separate set of staff nurses. With
a few exceptions, I believe it is a mistake for all concerned;
but I may well take this opportunity of impressing upon you
the importance of the duties and of the responsibilities which
rest in the hands of night nurses. The punctual administration
of food and medicine—the careful observation of symptoms
upon the immediate treatment of which life may depend—
the living and the dying are literally left in charge of the
night nurses, and are often, too, wholly dependent upon them.
It is a *great trust*, and I should like to have the comfort of
feeling that all of you thoroughly realize this, in order that
you may spare no effort to make yourselves worthy of it.

Those of you who may have read that beautiful poem of
Mrs. Hamilton King, "The Disciples," cannot fail to have
been struck with that wonderful "Sermon in the Hospital."
I am particularly glad to learn that it has now been published
separately from the complete volume, and is to be had as a
small pamphlet. I make this known to you, because I think
all nurses would be the better for reading it, and would
probably find their sympathy with suffering increased; and
I refer to it especially at this moment for the sake of two
lines there applied to the sick, but which night nurses may
well refer to themselves, and find help in the thought—

> "God gives His angels charge of those who sleep,
> But He Himself watches with those who wake."

Often and often I think of this when I have finished my
round of the wards, and go to bed fully realizing the long,
anxious watch before some of you. We know that a very

real blessing rests upon all loyal, faithful service; and I only remind you of it that you may do your work in such a way as to make this blessing your own.

> " The noblest service comes from nameless hands,
> And the best servant does his work unseen."

I have to-night attempted to point out the chief duties of a nurse in connection with the treatment of complete general rest, when it is ordered for a patient under her care. I speak of very small details, because it is these which might not otherwise occur to you; and yet the omission of them would at once show an experienced observer that you were not doing these simple, every-day duties with that finish which should characterize every item of a trained nurse's work.

Next time we will consider what a nurse has to keep in remembrance in connection with " partial rest," as supplied by splints, bandages, mechanical supports, and other local appliances, in carrying out that system of treatment.

LECTURE III.

THROUGHOUT all these lectures, I am anxious that you should keep in your mind the leading idea that nurses are active agents in carrying out a scientific system of treatment laid down by the doctor. I want you to look at your work from this point of view, because I am confident that it will be of service, both in showing what your own line is, and what are its limits, and also in helping you to keep to them.

I told you last time that treatment presents itself to us under one or more of the three following aspects. First, to provide an antidote to any poison, and to remove all sources of harm; as, for instance, in removing a person who was suffering from the ill effects of an infected neighbourhood to a healthy locality, or giving up an occupation which produced disease. Secondly, to put the patient in the most favourable position for self-cure; as, in the breaking of a fractured limb, at rest in the right position, and leaving Nature to effect her own cure without interruption. Thirdly, to aid in treatment by drugs which experience or experiment have shown to be efficacious—as in the case of certain applications for skin disease—which may be all the treatment needed. I endeavoured to explain that one of these methods of treatment may suffice—as in the illustrations I have just given you—or that a combination of all three may be desirable —as in a case of rheumatic fever, for instance, when it would be necessary to remove the patient from all influences considered to be conducive to rheumatism, whether it was the locality in which the patient lived, or the kind of work in which he was engaged. During an acute attack of rheumatic fever, it would be necessary to keep the patient in a suitable temperature at rest in bed between blankets; to give suitable diet; and, finally, to aid in the treatment by such drugs as the doctor might consider most likely to be beneficial to the case; and thus all three methods of treatment would be employed. The more you reflect on the subject for yourselves, the more clearly you will see that all treatment does present itself to us under one or more of these aspects.

You are aware, also, that when we speak of therapeutics we mean treatment; and that treatment consists in the application of natural agents, such as rest, cold, heat, and others too numerous for us to enter into now. We divided the first of these into two headings—*general* rest, as applied to the whole body, whether complete or comparative; and *partial* rest, as it is prescribed in the form of splints, bandages, and other mechanical supports, to meet local emergencies.

We fully entered into the first half of the subject last time, and to-night we will first turn our attention to the details it is desirable you should know in connection with the second part of this subject; and this brings us to the question of partial rest, as supplied by splints, bandages, and strapping.

I do not propose to weary you with verbal descriptions of the different kinds of splints, the names and patterns for various purposes used in this and in other hospitals; these can be learned best in the wards; neither have I forgotten that in the course of another two or three months you will be having the benefit of most interesting and useful lectures on "Surgical Nursing." But there are a few small points that surgeons seldom remember to mention; perhaps they fancy that a knowledge of them comes intuitively to nurses, though we all know this is not quite the case.

It is especially the nurses' business to take pains with the cleansing and padding of splints. There are innumerable kinds of splints made of various materials—wood, metal, gutta percha, leather, and other new and improved materials are constantly being introduced. In cases of emergency, broomstick handles sawn in two, and newspapers, have served the purpose when nothing else was to be had. I once heard of an old copy of the *Times* newspaper being folded up· and used most successfully as the splint for a fractured humerus by a skilful surgeon, when the accident happened far from civilized regions, and no better appliance could be obtained. I mention this, though, merely as an interesting incident, not with the anticipation that you will ever be expected to prepare newspaper splints. The names of the splints most used for their respective purposes, and the comparative advantages and disadvantages of different kinds—any special points to remember in the padding of any of them—are all matters for practical experience in the wards, and it is only in this way that the requisite knowledge can be acquired. To give you minute theoretical instruction on these details would be an utter waste of time, so I shall confine my remarks on the subject to a few general and important statements.

You can scarcely be too careful about cleansing and disinfecting *all* splints that are to be used again. Never put them away dirty by any chance, and think you will attend to them when you have more time, and that it will be all right if you can manage to get them ready somehow before they are wanted. They may be wanted suddenly, when perhaps you are not there ; and it is infinitely better that you should have the extra trouble of cleaning them again, if they have time to get soiled before they are wanted, than that any risk should be run of infecting a patient by the application of a splint that is not absolutely clean. I need scarcely point out to you how readily the contagion of erysipelas or pyæmia may be conveyed from one patient to another by an uncleansed or inefficiently cleansed splint. It is not too much to say that lives may be, and, unfortunately, have been, lost, solely through the carelessness—I may fairly say, the unconscientious carelessness—of nurses indifferent to, or ignorant of, the danger. After all, ignorance is not a very adequate excuse, if we hold a position which makes us, under certain conditions, responsible for the lives of some of our fellow-creatures. It is terrible that some are sacrificed mainly through such avoidable causes. The more we think of the responsibility attaching to a nurse's work, the more vividly we must realize the grave importance of understanding as much as we can about everything we have to do, and the reason why these apparent trifles demand so much care and attention. Put plenty of carbolic acid in the water with which you cleanse splints, whether the case for which they have previously been used makes you think this precaution specially necessary or not.

Now, with regard to the padding of splints, as far as possible, you must take pains to pad to suit the ideas of the surgeon for whom you are working. Some give the preference to rather thick pads, some like them much thinner; all expect to have them *evenly* made, one of the objects in using them being to apply *equal* pressure. Soft old linen is the best material for covering pads, but as large hospitals are but insufficiently supplied with this, we are obliged to use unbleached calico. Some prefer making the entire pad of blanket; but this material is not conducive to cleanliness, as you will soon perceive for yourselves if you ever have them used in wards in which you are working. A mixture of tow and wool is generally used to stuff pads. All wool is said not to have sufficient "spring" in it, besides being extravagant. Tow is not sufficiently soft to be employed alone. All lumps must be carefully avoided, whatever material is used. Nothing

E

can be more admirably adapted to its purpose than the padding
wool sold especially for it. It is very expensive, but it is
excellent; and in using it you must combine economy with
extreme care not to run the slightest risk for the patients, by
making up pads with a single morsel of padding wool that is
not as safe for the purpose as that which comes straight out
of a new packet.

In many cases pads are covered with gutta percha tissue,
though this occasionally irritates the skin. The object of
waterproof covering for splints is to keep them clean and
dry, notwithstanding applications of a moist and greasy
nature. Oiled cotton can also be used, and it does not
produce the irritating effect of gutta percha tissue, but the
disadvantage of it is that it is not very soft to place next the
skin. One point you should be careful to remember in
padding all kinds of splints, and that is to make the pads
sufficiently large to thoroughly cover the sides of the splints,
and not leave the hard edges without this protection. If
any surgeon objects to this, you must at once endeavour to
meet his wishes, but such objection will be the exception and
not the rule. The pads should be sewn on with long even
stitches, but if they are wanted in great haste or if additional
pads are suddenly required—as they sometimes are in the
operating theatre, for instance—a piece of strapping quickly
wound across will serve to keep them in place admirably. In
applying or helping others to apply splints always have cotton
wool at hand; it is often serviceable in preventing or
relieving pressure. If patients complain of much pain after
the application of splints, be sure and notice if there is much
swelling or discoloration of the adjacent parts, and call the
sister's attention to it at once; though of course you would
not think of loosening the bandage on your own responsibility.

Plaster of Paris, starch, gum and chalk, silicate of potass,
applied with bandages are light forms of splints that you

will often see put on in the wards. They keep an injured joint in position in a form least inconvenient to the patient when he begins to move about. A flannel or domette bandage will always be applied to the limb before the other, and some cotton wool is frequently required. I will not enter into further details of how to prepare these, as you will all be able to learn it better practically in the wards. If patients are going about much with these splints on, the white of an egg painted on as a varnish is useful to prevent chipping. Sand-bags are extremely useful to keep injured limbs still and in position ; they should be made of tick, such as is employed for making beds, because it is strong and close in texture, and sand is very heavy. The sand-bags should then be covered with mackintosh, oiled cotton, or gutta percha tissue, to keep them dry and clean, and finally it is a refinement of nursing to cover them with little cases of unbleached calico that are made to come on and off as pillow cases do ; they are then ready to be supplied clean for each patient, or whenever necessary, and look neat and " finished " in the bed. Be sure in making sand-bags that the sand is thoroughly dry.

Strapping is applied to various parts of the body by way of affording support and even pressure. The strapping should be carefully ruled before cutting to ensure evenness, and the strips must be cut the required length and width. The nurse must be quick and attentive in handing the surgeon the strips as he is ready for them, duly warmed by placing the non-adhesive side of the plaster across the hot water strapping tins. Some surgeons prefer the strapping dipped into hot water, but they will tell you so in these instances, for this is exceptional, and the other method is far cleaner and nicer for adoption as a general rule. Fractured ribs are frequently treated by strapping the chest, to afford support and secure the greatest possible "rest" to the injured part. With some surgeons strapping is a favourite form of treatment for ulcerated legs, and this reference reminds me to tell you that when you are ordered to remove strapping from wounds, you must be extremely careful not to drag open the wound. In removing strapping from wounds you should begin at both ends and work towards the centre of the wound. This is an important point to remember, not only for the sake of avoiding pain to the patient, but to prevent all risk of breaking down or injuring any union that may be taking place. An ignorant nurse removing strapping roughly and clumsily may during the process undo the work of weeks, so please do not regard this as a trifling detail.

If it falls to your share to apply strapping to an ulcerated leg, remember you stand in front of your patient in the same way that you would to put on a bandage. Then pass the well-warmed strip of plaster under the limb, and apply the middle of it to the back of the leg, bringing the ends round the sides of the leg and crossing them over in front. Each succeeding strap should overlap its predecessor about one third of its width. I dare say most of you have seen how neat it can be made to look if it is skilfully done.

The strapping put on the leg to enable extension to be applied is often left to the nurse to do. A practical illustration of how it is done is better than a verbal description. You must be careful to put on the strapping in such a way as to avoid wrinkles, and as far as possible to avoid pressure sores. This point needs a great deal of attention, and you must always see carefully if anything is wrong when the patient complains of pain in this respect. A little piece of wool under the heel or between the loose part of the strapping may often save a great deal of suffering. It is a good plan to cut a small hole in the loose part of the strapping for extension, which comes over the ankle to relieve all chance of pressure or friction there. Small pieces of lint should be neatly wound round the foot to prevent all avoidable discomfort, and infinite pains must be taken to make every arrangement possible for the patient not to suffer any un-necessary inconvenience, nor to run any risk of the treatment of extension having to be given up in consequence of external sores. Remember the weight must not be put on until the strapping has had time to adhere firmly. A flannel bandage is put on over the strapping. When the extension has been applied you must lift the weights carefully before giving the patient the bed-pan.

You must never ignore a patient's complaints of a splint or piece of strapping being too tight. The sores which come in consequence are often difficult to heal. Take care that the sister knows of the complaint, that she may attend to it. Of course you must not alter anything the surgeon has applied without orders to do so. After plaster of Paris and other bandages of the same description, swelling is apt to take place, and you must notice if the part below the bandage swells or becomes discoloured. Some patients will complain of the least discomfort, and others are too patient to complain readily, so a nurse must be watchful on these points.

To get off the dirty marks of strapping use a little oil; turpentine, of course, is effectual, but that is rather harsh; chloroform is also excellent for the purpose, but you would not be likely to have it about for general use in the wards, and it should be remembered that chloroform blisters some skins.

I may as well mention also that strapping is cut in a special manner for cases of hare-lip. I should scarcely succeed in conveying to you a clear idea of the arrangement merely by a verbal description. You must take the earliest opportunity of getting a practical illustration in the wards, and any private nurse who finds herself obliged to undertake a case of hare-lip without previous experience should remember to ask the surgeon how he wishes the strapping cut before the operation begins.

Another method of cutting strapping is useful in cases where it is desirable to afford support and at the same time to keep an outlet for the discharge. This is known as grid-iron strapping, a portion of the strapping being cut into strips in a manner suggestive of the name.

When antiseptic dressings have to be kept in place with strapping some surgeons prefer that the strips shall be moistened by dipping them into a hot solution of carbolic acid (1 to 19) instead of warming them in the usual way.

Arm, leg, and general bed-rests of various kinds must be adjusted to suit each case in the manner that will be shown to you in your practical work, and you must apply such common sense and intelligence as you are fortunate enough to possess, to the complete understanding of the principle and skilful adjustment of such appliances. I should mention in connection with the use of bed-rests that the tendency which weak patients have to slip down in the bed when the upper part of the body is raised against a bed-rest is frequently a source of discomfort, and the convenient, in-expensive footpiece, with pieces of webbing attached to enable it to be graduated in conjunction with the bed-rest to the needs of the patient, which has been invented by Mr. Newton Nixon, of University College Hospital, seems likely to prove of great service.

The application of slings is frequently left to the nurse, without any special directions being given; so there are two or three facts in connection with their adjustment that it may be useful to you to know.

In injuries to the arm or hand, in nearly every case, the sling should support the whole of the forearm, including the elbow. The only exception to this would be a fracture of the upper arm, in which case the pushing up of the elbow would have a tendency to displace the fracture, and it is better to employ a narrow sling for the wrist or hand only.

To support the foot, the sling should be placed round the neck. For slinging up the arm or foot in a recumbent position, webbing should be attached at intervals to the cradle, which is placed over the injured limb to relieve the pressure of the bedclothes. With regard to the varying height at which it should be slung up, I can only recommend you to carefully note how the surgeon places the limb when he slings it up in the first instance, and endeavour to keep it in exactly the same position.

A three-cornered bandage can be used advantageously as a sling, and it can also be adapted with excellent effect to most purposes for which ordinary bandages are applied. This is called the Esmarch bandage, from the name of the inventor. You must get taught in the wards the various methods in which they can be applied.

This leads us up to the subject of bandages—one of universal interest to nurses. I only propose to-night to deal with the theory of bandaging; that is, to lay before you certain fixed principles for you to keep in your mind as a guide for the practical work.

I am anxious to point out to you that it rests much more with yourselves than you appear to think to attain proficiency in bandaging. You hope to learn that amongst other nursing accomplishments; but how, where, and when, probationers leave to circumstances in a manner that is, I think, rather disappointing, and certainly unwise for yourselves.

I do not attach much value to bandaging classes, because, as every learner cannot receive individual attention at once, it entails considerable waste of time, and there is no single advantage to be gained by them that cannot equally be obtained in the wards.

I most strongly recommend you to avoid *practising* on lay figures and blocks, if you wish to become good bandagers. The sensation—if one may so speak—of handling stiff, unyielding material, however well shaped to the limb, is so different to the comparatively elastic touch of living muscle, that my observation in this matter has led me to the conclusion that practising bandaging on lay figures is not only undesirable, but harmful. This is my opinion on the subject, and it is due to you that I should put before you the result of my experience; but I need scarcely say that you are not bound to adopt my convictions for your own. At the same time, I would not be understood as condemning the practice of being shown the manner of applying any particular bandage, or of just learning the actual method of the application on a lay figure yourself. The custom I deprecate is *practising*, with a view of obtaining proficiency, on a lay figure, under the impression that it is as satisfactory for the purpose as a living subject.

Choose your opportunities of practising and of being shown, but *look out* for them, and do not wait, as children might do, for others to be more anxious to teach you than you are to learn. If you are eager to learn, and exercise a little discretion in the time when you ask to be taught, you will find no lack of ready and skilful teachers. Many of you could improve the time when you have what we are apt to call an uninteresting special case on your hands, by practising on any good-natured convalescent patient, who is inclined to be amused at the proceeding, or on another nurse or probationer, who may have a few minutes to spare. I know that for the most part your time is closely filled up, but I am confident that every one of you will find innumerable opportunities if you care to take the trouble. Some of you on night duty waste valuable time and chances in wards where there are two of you on duty, and there are occasional, if rare, half-hours when your patients are wanting nothing; and it is pleasant to me to know that nowhere could you find night sisters more cordially interested in and desirous of helping you.

Of course, put your patients and your work for them *first*
—a long way first—but do not forget that self-improvement
in the branch of education that you have come here to study
is also a 'duty that you have no right to neglect. I do not
want you to become more selfish, but I should like to see the
majority of you a degree more eager to " train yourselves."
I say this without reservation, having too much confidence
in you to fear that you will misinterpret my meaning. Nothing
but constant practice can perfect you in any mechanical
accomplishment; and I simply want to put before you that,
if you cannot take the personal trouble necessary, you must
inevitably remain more or less ignorant. You must not
imagine that bandaging is only to be thought of in surgical
wards. On the contrary, you had better practise on sound
than on injured limbs. When you have to take the latter in
hand, it is well you should know how to manage them.

Now that I have said so much, perhaps I had better
mention that I am not desirous of this kind of thing being
done too obtrusively and at all seasons in the wards. I should
be sorry to come across visions of probationers bandaged up
by each other in all directions, and for you to be under the
impression that this was my wish ! I have not had sufficient
evidence of energy in this respect. My impression is, that
the idea of *getting yourselves taught* bandaging has not
occurred to many of you, and I hope now that many will act
on my suggestion; only do not go to the other extreme.
Most nurses are, or should be, familiar with Berkeley Hill's
work on the " Essentials of Bandaging," and I am glad to
quote some of his clear and condensed instructions to you
to-night.

Bandages are made of ordinary flannel, domette, unbleached calico, linen, muslin, or gauze of various kinds. In
preparing them for use, remember that selvages must *always*
be removed, and, of course, avoid joins as much as possible.

Where economy or any other reason necessitates them, be
sure to make the seam as flat and smooth as possible, and
do not use big knots in your cotton. All bandages must be
rolled tightly, to enable them to be satisfactorily applied.
The lengths vary from six to twelve yards, generally some
length between these two measurements. It is not a proof
of good bandaging to see how much bandage you can wind
on, but rather, within certain limits, to ascertain how little
will answer the purpose satisfactorily, without cumbering the
limb unnecessarily. At the same time, it is often essential to
extend the bandage considerably beyond the exact spot which
renders its application necessary, to prevent the swelling of
adjacent parts. Endeavour to understand as far as possible
with what object the bandage is ordered. It may be merely
to secure a dressing being kept in place ; it may be to supply
firm support ; it may be to check hemorrhage, or for some
other reason. But, in any case, remember to keep the primary
object in view, whatever that may be ; next, have due regard
to the comfort of the patient; and, finally, to the neat appearance of your bandage. Bandages are of various widths,
according to the purpose for which they are required.

Head-rollers	are usually about	2 inches wide
Arm-rollers	,, ,,	$2\frac{1}{4}$,,
Leg-rollers	,, ,,	3 ,,
Rib or chest rollers	., ,,	6 ,,
Toe or finger rollers	,, ,,	only $\frac{3}{4}$ or $\frac{1}{2}$ an inch.

Occasionally double-headed rollers are required, i.e., the
bandage is rolled up from both ends towards the centre, so
that you have, as it were, two rollers joined together to work
with. This is convenient for the capeline and some other
bandages.

When you are going to apply a bandage, place yourself
opposite the patient, not by the side. Always make a firm
and fixed beginning for a starting-point, not on the place for

which the bandage is needed, but beneath. "When applying a roller, it is best to begin by placing the outer surface
of the roller next the skin. . . . The bandage should be
carried from the inner side of the limb by the front to the
outer side." Bandage upwards. The turns must never be
made over a prominence of bone. There are three different
turns, the simple spiral, the reverse, and the figure of eight.
The spiral bandage is sufficient when both edges of bandage
can lie evenly on the surface of the limb, but when the limb
enlarges too fast for this, the turn must be interrupted, and
brought back by a reverse ; or, if over a joint, for instance,
by figure of eight.

At the moment of reversing, hold the bandage quite
loosely, and the thumb of the unoccupied hand must fix the
lower border of the bandage at the highest point of the turn,
while the roller is turned over in the other hand and passed
downwards to overlap the previous turn evenly. All the
reverses must be carried one above the other, along the
outer side of the limb, and only employed when necessary.

Figures of eight are made exactly as their name implies,
by passing the roller alternately upwards and downwards as it
enwraps the limb. They are adopted where the enlargement
is too great and irregular for reverses to lie evenly, as the
ankle, the elbow, or the knee. It is of the first importance
that bandages should be adapted to the object for which they
are employed, whatever that may be. They must not be too
tight over dressings. They must afford steady, *even* pressure,
and not be tight and loose alternately.

To get reverses always outside limbs, you must learn to
bandage with both hands with equal facility. But do not
make turns over a wound when it can possibly be avoided ;
for instance, if the ulcer is on the outside of the leg, make
your reverses inside, avoiding the prominence of bone. The
patient must always be the *first* consideration, and every other

nursing quality comes *after* that. Nothing but constant practice can teach you how to do the various kinds of bandages with skill, neatness, and finish. It rests with all probationers who pass through our training school to maintain the reputation of being good bandagers for London hospital nurses.

The T bandage is made with two pieces of bandage, the end of one joined to the centre of the other, which should be long enough to tie round the waist and fasten in front; the other end should reach from the centre of the back, under the perinæum, and up to the waist in front. This piece may be left entire or slit into two tails, which can be fastened separately over each groin. This is a most useful bandage for keeping applications in place.

The same may be said of four-tailed, six-tailed, and many-tailed bandages. These are made by joining the requisite number of strips of bandage, slightly overlapping each other, on to a central piece of bandage. The particular advantage of the many-tailed bandage for those cases to which they are applicable is that the dressings can be changed without moving the limb, and thus much pain, and possibly some increase of injury, may be spared to the patient.

The capeline bandage for the head is not infrequently used, and is serviceable occasionally. There is nothing specially to mention in the theory of its application, and you must try and get practical illustrations of it and individual practice in applying it in the wards.

The single and double spica bandage is a figure of eight applied to one or both groins.

A bandage for the jaw has a small slit made lengthways in the centre to support the chin, and the ends are slit a little way down, so as to fasten partially at the back of the head and partially at the top, as this serves to keep it in place.

Rib rollers are the best kind of bandage with which to apply jacket poultices, but a broad piece of calico, rather

more than the depth of the poultice, brought from under the
back, and fastened with strings or safety pins in front, and
with two strips of bandage sewn at the top of both sides at
the back, and brought over the shoulders, to fasten with
safety pins in front, will keep the poultice securely in position,
and be less fatiguing for the patient when the poultice is
renewed than the rolling and unrolling of a bandage on each
occasion. This reminds me to tell you that in taking off a
bandage you should gather it promptly up in your hands as
fast as you unwind it, and not leave it hanging loose, to drag
more or less by the yard, as you remove it. I think there is
nothing else of importance for me to tell you about the
principles of bandages. I can only hope that you will all
endeavour to become proficient in practice.

I will take this opportunity of making a few observations
to you on the subject of surgical dressings generally. I am
aware that, strictly speaking, they can scarcely be considered
under the heading of partial rest, the question to which we
are turning our attention to-night; but in the practical part
of a nurse's work the preparation and application of dressings
is very closely allied to that of splints and bandages, so I
think that such a digression is not unpardonable.

When I speak of surgical dressings, I do not mean that I
am going to tell you minutely why various dressings are
used, what are the various characteristic appearances of
different wounds, nor what is implied by the well-known
expressions commonly used in reference to them, for this wide
subject will be duly set before you in detail in the course of
lectures which will immediately follow mine ; but the points
I wish to speak of in connection with this subject are those
which surgeons commonly take for granted that nurses know
by instinct, or which they have never happened to notice
themselves.

I need scarcely tell you that no amount of theoretical

instruction will be of the same value as the practice you get daily in the wards; but I am confident that a combination of theory with the practical experience you are now gaining will not only enable you to learn better, but to learn quicker, because you will be able to profit to the utmost by what you see and hear, instead of carrying out the duties which fall to your share quite mechanically. Of course do what you are told *with implicit obedience*, whether you understand the object with which the orders are given or not; but the more you understand, the better it will be for yourselves and all concerned, provided, of course, that you are careful never to obtrude your knowledge.

I am anxious that in teaching you, and in every arrangement made for your efficient training, you shall know *fully* everything which a good nurse ought to know and do in every branch of your profession; but I am also most anxious that you should carefully guard against every temptation to display that knowledge, *except practically*. The perfection for a nurse is to know everything that she is wanted and expected to know, and to let every one under whom she works be able to safely take it for granted that she possesses the requisite knowledge. It is never necessary for a nurse to say, "I can do this and that," or "I think this and that," unless she is asked the direct question. The golden rule for nurses to remember is to "state facts, not opinions," and I pause to remind you of this, because we are more likely to fall into this error when our knowledge is comparatively new, as it is with probationers, than when we have become so familiar with nursing details that we can scarcely believe there was ever a time when we did not know them. I want you each to cultivate for *yourselves* any little habit of finish or neatness that I may now speak of, so that from sheer custom it would be awkward for you to do things in any other way. By-and-by, you will wonder that you ever needed to be told of them, only it will be your turn to teach others then, I hope, and you will see over again that a knowledge of nursing does not come instinctively, and will, I trust, be patient and painstaking when it becomes your turn to teach.

In a surgical ward, when the general work is straight, the next thing a nurse has to think about is getting the dressings ready. There are so many different dressings in different degrees of favour with different surgeons, that it would be impossible to speak of all of them in detail. A nurse should endeavour that every case should have the dressing needed for it waiting by the bed for the dresser or the house surgeon. In an efficient ward they should never have to wait, except when such fresh things are wanted that a nurse could not be supposed to know about them beforehand. Of course in children's wards you will take care that the waiting dressings are not left within their reach. It is either laziness or great want of thought on the part of a nurse to wait until the dressings are asked for, because "perhaps they won't be wanted," or they are " not quite sure that ' the dressing ' will be done to-day." That is a slovenly sort of way for a nurse to get into, and I am always sorry when I hear of any instance of the kind. Besides, uncertainty as to what the surgeon or dresser may decide to do, does not alter the fact that it is a nurse's business to have everything in her department quite ready. Of course, if you are uncertain what to do, ask the sister, or, if she gives you any direction, you have only to follow it ; but whilst I am most particular that you should always refer to the sister, and not take things upon yourselves, I am afraid you often make her work heavier than it need be by throwing upon her the responsibility of reminding you of every little thing. There is great scope for careful observation in this getting ready of dressings, and any trouble you take in this respect will repay you greatly.

In doing dressings yourselves be quite sure that you have everything ready before you begin. It does not matter how long or how short a time you may have been in a hospital, but you cannot consider yourselves "trained" while you find that you have to leave off in the middle and fetch what you knew beforehand you would require if you had only troubled to think about it. You will need an empty receiver ready for the soiled dressings. I have been surprised before now to see these soiled dressings thrown about on the sheet, the check, or even the floor, just because the receiver was not at hand for the purpose. It does not save trouble, for, of course, they have to be picked up again, and it is obviously a very objectionable and dirty arrangement.

Each of you should provide yourselves with a pair of dressing forceps, scissors, and pins, and be sure you accustom yourselves to use the forceps, and not your fingers, for touching those dressings which are in contact with the wound or soiled with discharge. I have already warned you as forcibly as I can on the subject of covering up your fingers if you have the very tiniest pin prick on them. You all know how quickly the worst forms of poison may be taken into the system in this way, and I can only repeat my former injunction, and remind you that a nurse cannot be too careful of her hands. You must also be extremely cautious not to put your fingers to your face, or eyes, or mouth, when you are doing dressings, until you have washed your hands.

In some hospitals it is the custom to use the irrigator for washing wounds ; in some the glass syringe ; in some an ordinary syringe with a glass nozzle fitted on to go in the wound, and in some hospitals these are only used when the house surgeon orders it, and other cases are washed with tow, cotton wool, lint, or linen. The one thing which should never be used for this purpose is a sponge, because of the difficulty of effectually cleansing it. For private cases the objection to this is lessened, because, as you would be using this for one case only, there would be no risk of taking any poison from one wound to another, and, of course, you would keep it soaking in some disinfectant; but when you have accustomed yourselves to using little pieces of cotton wool, you will certainly prefer it. I must not forget to speak of the way in which this should be done. Nearly all wounds now are cleansed with warm water, to which a little carbolic lotion has been added. Now there cannot be any necessity for dipping the piece of cotton wool which is soiled with discharge into the basin or the receiver which contains the water that you are using for this purpose, and thus soiling the whole of the contents. The next time you wipe round the wound, neither the wool nor the water will be perfectly clean. You should take a little piece of wool, soak it in and wring it out of this water, and when you have used it, put it in the receiver which contains the soiled dressings, and take a fresh little bit of wool each time until you have finished the washing. Small pieces of soft old rag will answer the purpose equally well if you have a supply of them.

For washing a wound you should place a dressing tray or a small basin, whichever appears more convenient, under the limb, so that there may be no difficulty in keeping the bed and the patient dry, and very often a mackintosh may be wanted for the purpose also. In washing wounds avoid *touching the edges*, as that gives the most pain. Wash *round* them gently and firmly *towards* and *not away from* the centre of the wound, and if it is necessary to touch the surface do it lightly. You will remove the stains of ointment, etc., best by a quick circular movement, and the marks of strapping can be removed with a little oil or turpentine, as I have just observed; but be sure, if you need to use the latter, you keep it carefully away from the wound. Never let your

F

patients be more exposed than is absolutely necessary for doing the dressing; see that they are comfortably covered up, and not risking cold. The wound must *never* be left uncovered. If you are cleaning it preparatory to a poultice, cover it up with a little piece of wet lint or linen while you are making the poultice, and see that the windows are closed. For a recent wound cold water, sometimes iced water, is used for cleansing it, for fear of renewing the tendency to bleed, but for wounds of longer date, warm water is generally used, as I said before. In removing strapping, I may remind you again here, that you must take great care that you do not undo much of the good that may have been done by pulling the edges of the wound open. You should begin to take it off first at one end until you come near the wound, then at the other, and finally with a little care you will be able to remove it without hurting the wound in any way. When you can, put the finger of one hand on the skin from which you are removing the strapping, so that there may be no "tearing sensation" for the patient. Never remove dressings roughly when they are adherent to a wound. They often become very stiff with blood and discharge, but you must thoroughly saturate them with lukewarm water or oil, so as to avoid tearing open the wound or breaking down any union which may have taken place. You must be very gentle in doing this, not only to prevent hurting the patient, but for fear of the harm you may do by any carelessness in this respect. When ointments or some liquid dressings are ordered to be applied to sores, you must remember it is useless to apply them over hard dry scabs. These must first be removed, and the process of getting them off will be much facilitated by the free application of oil, which softens them. Remember that forceps, not fingers, must be used for the purpose. Always keep the hair cut quite close near any wound or sore place, or it will interfere in many ways with the dressing. Be sure in dressing burns that you do not expose the whole or much of an injured surface at one time. The old dressings must be removed and the new ones replace them by very careful degrees, not all at once.

Nurses in this hospital have seldom much to do with preparing large quantities of zinc dressing, but in private nursing it would fall to their share, therefore I may as well mention that it will greatly facilitate the process of spreading the ointment if you dip the spatula frequently into hot water. The grease of the ointment of course will not mix with the water, and the hot blade of the spatula will spread it more quickly and smoothly. Zinc dressings should always be kept ready spread, and nurses should not get into the habit of putting a little ointment on a piece of lint just when it is required. It is wasteful, and the application is not in such good condition. When you are told to apply zinc or any other stimulating dressing, you must remember that it is intended the application should be the *exact* size of the wound, *not spread over the edges*, as may be done with oil or simple dressing, and cover it with a layer of a larger piece of lint or linen spread with some non-irritating ointment. You will soon learn for yourselves in the wards to what other applications this rule applies.

Scott's dressing, which is a harder substance to spread than zinc ointment, should always be kept by the nurse spread on lint and cut into strips ready for use. It is usually ordered to be applied to joints, *i.e.*, strips of the dressing wound over the joint and then covered with strips of strapping. Water dressings and some lotions (not evaporating) should be applied on a piece of lint folded double and covered with a piece of gutta percha tissue or oiled silk, which should be cut a little larger than the dressing so as to completely cover it.

In most hospitals, and this amongst the number, lint is

used with the plain side towards the patient, and ointments
are spread upon that side. In some books, however, you will
find directions to the contrary, so if you are told to use it in
that way, you need not look upon it as an unheard-of thing.
Your best plan is always to follow the custom of the hospital
in which you are working; both ways are right, inasmuch as
they have been approved by good authorities who happened
to differ on the subject.

Carbolic oil or oiled lint, as it is generally called in the
wards, should be wrung out very dry and kept in stock
ready for use. When these dressings are wanted they should
always be cut ready for the purpose and put neatly in the
dressing trays, so that they can be readily handed to the
surgeon, and that they may not soil the bedclothes or any
place on which they may be put.

I believe that this is all I have to say to you in connection
with these details.

LECTURE IV.

Now we come to the consideration of cold and heat as remedial
agents, their respective properties as such, and then their
varied forms of application. Cold and heat are relative
terms, and are used in a comparative sense. Temperature is
a state of matter, a condition in which matter is; not matter
itself. Our original ideas of cold and heat are influenced by
the temperature of our bodies. If a substance is of lower
temperature than ourselves, we call it cool or cold, according
to the degree of difference which exists, and in the same way
we call any substance of a higher temperature than ourselves
warm or hot. A cold substance is warm compared to one
cooler than itself, and a hot substance is cool compared to
one hotter than itself. That is what I mean by saying that
cold and heat are relative terms. For instance, ice is water,
i.e., matter in a state of cold called freezing; steam is water,
i.e., matter in a state of evaporation. This single illustration
will serve to show you what I mean by temperature being
a state of matter.

Living things produce heat; or, to put it more forcibly, the
production of heat is a property of all living matter. The
animal heat of our bodies is of the same nature, and caused
in the same way as heat in a fire, that is, by the union of
oxygen with other substances. But I do not propose to enter
into the physiological aspects of the question, nor to say more
about temperature to-night. We will confine ourselves to the

properties of heat and cold, as remedial agents, and the objects for which they are thus employed. Heat and cold act by modifying the supply of blood to the surface, *i.e.*, by diminishing it, which is the effect produced by cold; by increasing it, which is the effect produced by heat. With this alteration in the quantity of blood goes also an alteration of sensibility, *i.e.*, diminished sensibility, as produced by cold up to complete loss of sensation; increased sensibility, as produced by heat up to scalding, with all the varied degrees of sensibility between these two extremes, such as the sensitiveness of a surface after the application of a poultice, or the coolness of a part to which an evaporating lotion has been applied.

The main uses of these natural agents, then, are: (1) to modify the amount of blood to the surface; (2) to reduce temperature; (3) to increase temperature.

They act as cold producers by direct abstraction of heat, by conduction, and by evaporation, thus producing a fall of temperature. I will explain more fully what we mean by these terms by-and-by.

They act as heat producers—(1) directly by the application of a hot substance; (2) indirectly by the diminution of evaporation, and so by preventing the fall of temperature.

Now, as a remedial agent cold is employed as a solid, as in the form of ice bags or Leiter's tubes, and as a liquid, as in the form of water and cooling lotions.

It is used for at least six distinct objects. (1) As a *stimulant* —in the way of dashing cold water over people in various methods. It is thus employed in cases of alcoholic poisoning, opium poisoning, or in recovering patients from the effects of chloroform, fainting, and so on. (2) It is used as a tonic— when employed with a view to producing reaction, as in the ordinary cold bath. (3) As an abstractor of heat—to reduce temperature, as in cold packs, evaporating lotions, and that

class of remedies. (4) As an anæsthetic—either for the purpose of soothing pain or to produce complete loss of sensation,
(5) As a styptic—to arrest hemorrhage internally or externally. (6) To cause contraction of parts, as in cases of
hernia, for instance.

You see that the effects of cold on the human body are
various, according to the way in which it is applied. Cold
water is frequently employed to abstract heat from the whole
surface of the body, or from some particular part of it, or to
induce general or local excitement or shock. It is also
employed to reduce fever and allay inflammation. On exposure to cold, increased oxidation of the tissues takes place,
as is demonstrated by the greatly increased quantities of
carbonic acid thrown off by the lungs. However, until you
know more physiology, it is not needful to enter fully into
these questions. You will not have to *prescribe* cold in any
form, only to *apply* it in such a manner as comes within the
province of a nurse's duties; but I want you to understand
the properties of cold as a distinct form of treatment, that
you may carry out such treatment intelligently, and understand more or less what is aimed at when it is prescribed.
A speedy immersion of the whole or any part of the body in
cold water will first give a sensation of shock and chill, local
or general, as the case may be, which is almost instantaneously
followed by a glowing exhilarating sensation. The next stage
after this is "depression." The cold bath is considered
bracing and very conducive to health when reaction follows.
But the ordinary cold bath, which is so useful as a means of
preserving health, is seldom ordered for hospital patients, and,
except to recommend its use strongly to yourselves, I need not
say much about it. The temperature varies from 70° to
50° Fahrenheit—below 50° it is very cold. A cold hip bath
is not infrequently ordered in conjunction with a hot foot-
bath, as feeble circulation in the extremities, if thus dealt

with, need not interfere with the satisfactory application of cold to other parts. Sometimes the invigorating effects of a cold bath are increased by the addition of sea-salt to the water.

When a cold bath is ordered, the patient should not remain in the water after the reaction sets in, for fear of the depression which may supervene if the bath is too prolonged. From three to five minutes is long enough for a patient to remain in a cold bath, when no special orders are given.

Ice baths for the purpose of reducing the temperature of the body are nearly always given under medical super-vision, and in any case you would only assist in giving them at first under the immediate direction of those more ex-perienced than yourselves. In some hospitals ice baths are much used for typhoid and other high-temperature diseases. The utmost care and discrimination is needed. Brandy is frequently administered to the patient whilst in the bath, and at any rate it must always be close at hand, with a measure-glass, spoon, and some water or milk, in case of its being suddenly called for.

If no special bath-gown is kept for the purpose, the patient, after having the night dress removed, should be wrapped in a sheet, and, as that will cling closely to the body when wet, it is well to leave one arm uncovered, that the person who is superintending may have no difficulty in getting at the pulse, which he or she may probably wish to feel all or most of the time.

Hot bottles, and often hot blankets, are sometimes asked for immediately after the bath, to counteract any symptoms of collapse that may ensue.

This is one of the many occasions when it is necessary for a nurse to exercise her common sense and powers of observa-tion, to see at once what is needed, and to do what she is told with quiet promptitude. A fussy, bustling, noisy person is intolerable at such a time, and the same may be said of a slow, unobservant woman, who cannot see what is wanted, nor do what she is told with the intelligent quickness which is expected from her.

Ice baths are not resorted to now quite so much as they were at one time. Cold sponging is employed much more frequently, and this devolves entirely upon the nurse. You must remember that it is not necessary to expose the whole body at the same time, that you must not make the bed damp and uncomfortable, and that you should do it gently, quickly, and *thoroughly*.

When ice-cold sponging is ordered without any special directions, do not let the process of sponging exceed ten minutes, for fear of shock to the patient. Tepid sponging may be made a more soothing process, and need not be hurried over in less than fifteen minutes if it is made rather pleasant than disturbing to the patient. The best way of drying patients after sponging is to dab each part as you finish sponging it with a soft towel. You must endeavour to make the whole process as little fatiguing as possible, as when this treatment is followed it usually involves frequent repetition.

Cold packing is useful in fevers and acute inflammatory diseases. The patient's clothes must be removed, and the whole body enveloped in a wet sheet; mackintoshes and blankets must be placed under and over the patient, and be closely tucked in. The pack should last from thirty to fifty minutes; longer, if necessary. This treatment is said to develop the rash, to greatly reduce the fever, to quiet the pulse, to render the skin moist and comfortable, and to abate the restlessness and wandering. It usually induces sleep.

In acute rheumatism, when the intense pain forbids the patient to be moved, you should pack the front of the body, and put a separate wet compress on each joint, changing the compress frequently. A compress consists of several folds of linen, with a piece of dry linen over it. For sore throats a cold compress is more effectual if it is covered up with oiled silk or gutta percha tissue. A wet compress placed over the eyes often induces sleep when other remedies fail. It is a simple remedy, which can nearly always be tried with safety.

Nurses must recognize the fact that if cold lotions and applications are ordered, they are intended *to be kept cold*, and must attend to them accordingly. Drip-pots, appliances that are familiar to any of you who have ever been in the accident wards, are an excellent means of keeping up a steady supply of cold lotion. They are simple to arrange, merely consisting of a small porringer, or basin secured by strapping to some convenient point over the part for which they are required ; strips of lint or flannel, with one end dipped in the fluid contained in the pot, and the other hanging over the side, will secure a steady drip of the liquid as long as there is any left in the vessel. The nurse must make a careful arrangement of the bed with mackintosh, and in some cases an earthenware receiver of some kind to receive the lotion as it trickles down ; but, having done this, she has only to recollect that the drip-pot will require to be kept constantly full. It is certainly the method of keeping up a constantly cold and moist application which gives least trouble to the nurse. I cannot say that they add to the neat appearance of the ward ; but this is no argument against their use, though it is a strong reason for nurses to exercise such ingenuity as they may be fortunate enough to possess in making them look as little untidy as possible.

If you are applying cold rags dipped in water or spirit lotion to the head or any inflamed surface where there is no wound, use two rags or handkerchiefs, that one may have time to cool perfectly in the lotion, ready to replace the warm one. If you want to keep a cold, moist application over a wound, do not wring out a soiled rag or piece of lint in the lotion. It is dirty both for yourself and the patient. Moisten the piece of lint by dabbing it freely and gently with a clean piece dipped in the lotion and taken out dripping, until it is desirable to remove the piece next the wound, and replace it by a fresh one altogether. Moist *cold* applications must *not* be dry and lukewarm—that is not a trustworthy carrying out of orders. I will not suppose that any of *you* would content yourselves with just having it right for the doctor, and deliberately neglecting it at other times, though I am sorry to say that I have known nurses who consider that sufficient. I want to impress upon you that you must not content yourselves with *meaning* to keep it right, "unless you forget." Nurses, if they are to be depended upon, *must* learn to remember, and carefulness in these details is not only important for yourselves, but absolutely essential to the welfare of your patients.

Ice is immensely used in medical, surgical, and obstetric cases, both externally and internally, as a convenient form of applying intense cold. It must be remembered that extreme cold applied to one part without intermission produces loss of sensation, and so acts as an anæsthetic ; if too prolonged, the part will die, and become gangrenous. The benumbed condition is preceded by a sensation of pain, which must be avoided by care in the application when ice is intended to act as a refrigerator, and not as an anæsthetic. Ice is employed to abstract heat, to allay imflammation, to check bleeding, to produce contraction, and to destroy sensation. Externally, it is usually ordered in the form of bags, or in the form of Leiter's tubes, which are now frequently employed for all parts of the body.

The use of ice bags as an effectual means of applying cold-treatment locally needs rather more care and attention than some nurses are inclined to think. If they are allowed to remain on when all the ice has melted, it is not only that they cease to be of service, but that they do positive harm, by inducing the reaction which, you all know, follows the removal of any cold application.

If you have not fresh ice ready, as it should be, it is better to remove the bag than to leave the bag of hot water applied to the part for which ice has been ordered; for directly the last piece of ice has melted, the temperature of the ice water will rise rapidly to that of the part with which it is in contact. Wet rags renewed frequently may be employed in the interval, if it is very important to keep up the treatment.

Ice bags should not be much more than half filled, and must be so arranged that the entire *weight* does not rest on the patient, though the *bag* does. This is easily accomplished, when the ice bags are needed for injured limbs, by tying 'the bags to the cradles placed over them, and, if they are properly arranged, this keeps them in excellent position. It is rather more difficult to keep them nicely applied to the head, partly on account of the frequent restlessness of the patient in cases where this remedy is prescribed, and partly because there is not usually anything able to bear the weight to which the ice bag can be attached, immediately over the patient's head. The little cords with the means of raising or lowering the bag, or moving it from side to side, which are used in the wards, serve admirably for the purpose in this hospital, where we have rods for the curtains; and when you have beds without, you must exercise your ingenuity and adapt it to the requirements of your patient as best you can.

Ice bags must not be placed next the skin, as the application of intense cold is painful, and a thin covering between the bag and the patient makes a vast difference in the comfort, and sometimes in the possibility of bearing it. It serves the twofold purpose of preventing frost-bite and of absorbing the moisture condensed on the surface of the ice bag. It is not necessary to put the usual piece of lint between when applying ice bags to the head, unless it is shaved or bald, as the thickness of the hair answers the same purpose. In the well-known " Handbook for Hospital Sisters," by Miss Florence Lees, she tells us that " Dr. Stokes considers that the best way of applying ice to the head is to place a smooth piece of ice, two or three inches long and one and a half broad, in a cup of soft sponge, and pass it round and round over the head. The sponge absorbs the water, and the pain of the cold is avoided. When the sponge is saturated, it is to be squeezed, and the ice replaced." This is not very applicable to the majority of cases in a hospital, but I consider it a valuable hint for private nurses, and it may sometimes be serviceable with bad cases that have special nurses, whose sole duty it is to attend to them. Ice bags for the head or limbs are convenient in the form of an ordinary bladder, or made of India rubber somewhat of that shape.

Small ice bags for the throat, eyes, forehead, etc., are best made for each case by the nurse, of gutta percha tissue fastened into the required shape with chloroform, which will dissolve and stick the edges of the bag together quite securely. A little practice is necessary to do this neatly, but no special skill, for it is perfectly simple. A nurse should endeavour to adapt the shape of these to each case. For instance, those that are wanted to pass under the chin are best rounded out a little, and quite as easily made.

The same bags can be used, *for the same patient,* two or three times if the ice is put in carefully. A double supply of these bags should be used, so that in removing one the other can be instantly replaced, and the patient is not disturbed twice. This is a greater consideration with small ice bags, inasmuch

as the ice melts quickly, and they have to be frequently
renewed. In changing these little bags when the ice has
dissolved, cut off the extreme end, and, after emptying out
the water, leave it to get *quite* cold before refilling it with ice.
The ice must, of course, be broken up into small pieces, to
make it as little uncomfortable as possible for the patient.
If ice bags cause persistent pain, always report it.

Many of you are already familiar with Leiter's tubes, an
invention for maintaining a steady supply of cold to almost
any part of the body for which it may be required. A pail
of iced water is placed above, or at any rate higher up than
the patient, from which a tube supplies the water to the
pliable tubes placed on the patient. When the iced water has
circulated through these it is conveyed by another tube to a
vessel placed ready to receive it. A nurse should see from
time to time that the water is flowing through properly, as
the tube is a little apt to get stopped up and become in-
effectual, until a vigorous "blow" up the tube puts it all
right again. A piece of lint must be placed between the
patient and the tubes for the same reason that it is employed
in the application of ice bags, and the pail containing the
iced water must be neatly covered round with flannel or some
other material to absorb the moisture which rapidly condenses on the outside of the pail and will otherwise drop on
the bed or the patient.

Ice is best broken by any instrument that has a very fine
point. For dividing small pieces noiselessly and quickly,
there is nothing better nor more convenient than a strong
needle. If you wish to break it without waking a patient,
you should place the piece to be divided in your hand, on
a small handkerchief or cloth, and it will scarcely make the
faintest sound.

Ice keeps best in large pieces, so never break it up into
small ones until required for use. When you have no

refrigerator, ice should be kept wrapped up in a dark place, and put in such a manner that the water may drip away from it as it dissolves, and none of the remaining ice stands in the water.

When ice is wanted for a patient to suck, it should not be put on the locker in a saucer, so that as it dissolves the remainder is kept in the water, and consequently melts faster than it otherwise would do. The best and readiest hospital arrangement for the purpose is to take a jam pot, and tie a little piece of *new* flannel or lint over the top, depressing it in the centre to make a convenient place for putting the ice in. An end of a rib bandage is often wide enough for the purpose, and it looks well if tied on with a morsel of scarlet or blue wool, which is generally to be had at a moment's notice in the wards. It looks all the better in the wards of those nurses who take the trouble to keep pieces in readiness, with the corners of the flannel rounded off and worked over with a little of the coloured wool, but of course this is an ornament, and not a necessity. A plain piece of flannel tied on with a bit of thread is all that is absolutely necessary for the purpose. The jar should stand in a saucer, so that any overflow of water may go into that, and not wet the top of the locker; the greater part of it will drop into the jar while the ice remains on the top of the flannel.

Ice is used internally to allay thirst, to check bleeding from the mouth, throat, stomach, or lungs, and to allay nausea and sickness. *Constant* sucking of ice is most efficacious for acute inflammation of tonsils ; also for the sore throat of scarlet fever. In some cases of diphtheria it is well for the patient to continue sucking it, if possible, till the disease has fairly declined. It *may* be given to most patients, and *must* be given to some. Children generally dislike it, because it makes their teeth ache. Some care is necessary in giving it to unconscious or delirious patients, lest it slip into the

trachea, and bring on a fit of choking. It may be given for
the sickness which so often follows the administration of
chloroform and ether, when the patient is sufficiently recovered. Ice taken internally has a tendency to cause con-
stipation, and consequently to check diarrhœa.

Two parts of finely powdered ice and one part of common
salt, forms an anæsthetic sufficient to freeze tissues. It will
cause vesication if applied too long, but will not do so under
six minutes. The ether spray is usually preferred now.

Ice bags are sometimes applied to the head in *delirium
tremens*, and for the convulsions of children. Spinal ice bags
are said to be invaluable for convulsions, and many other
purposes. The mode in which they act, and the various
ways of applying them for different objects, are much extolled
by Dr. Chapman. Amongst other results, he states that the
application of ice to the spine will speedily make cold feet
comfortably warm. I mention the fact, thinking it may
interest you to notice it next time you have an opportunity,
though it would be out of place to enter into the physiological
explanation of it which he gives.

This, I think, is all I have to bring to your notice in
reference to a nurse's duties in applying cold as a remedial
agent both general and local. There is rather more detail to
speak of in connection with the *local* applications of heat;
but I think I shall still have time to-night to speak of its
uses as a remedial agent, and of the manner in which it can
be employed as a means of *general* treatment.

All bodies have a certain heat. The terms " heat " and
"cold" are only relative, as I have previously told you. All substances which are hotter than their neighbouring bodies, tend
to give up their heat until equalization is reached. Bodies lose
heat by conduction, by radiation, and some by evaporation.
I need not take up your time by endeavouring to give you a
full explanation of these terms, but I think it is essential that

you should understand what is meant by the term " evaporation." " Evaporation is the passage of a fluid into a gaseous
state." You know that fluids are volatile in various degrees.
If you place a saucer of eau de Cologne and a saucer of water
in a room, you are most of you aware that the saucer which
contained the eau de Cologne would be dry first; *i.e.*, the
evaporation of the spirit will be much more rapid than that
of the water. Heat especially increases evaporation. If you
placed a lighted spirit lamp under either the saucer of eau
de Cologne or of the water, the evaporation would be much
quicker in both instances. During the process of evaporation
—*i.e.*, of the passage of a fluid into a gas or vapour—heat is
used up. This heat must come from somewhere, and it comes
from what is in the immediate neighbourhood, *i.e.*, from the
bodies nearest it.

Of course, for a body to lose heat by evaporation, it must
contain fluid, evaporation being defined as the passage of a
fluid into a gaseous state. Such bodies as do not contain fluid
can only lose heat by conduction and radiation. Our bodies
do contain fluid; therefore we lose heat, to some extent, by
conduction and by radiation, but evaporation is our chief
means of loss.

Now, our bodies produce heat and lose heat. I must not
linger to describe to you the manner in which we produce
heat, but I want you to grasp the fact that our mean temperature is the balance between the production of heat in
us and the loss of heat from us; and either the production
or the loss may be increased or diminished, and so the
temperature rises or falls. To be more explicit, if we produce
heat in excess, and do not lose heat in the same proportion,
our temperature rises; if we do not produce more than the
normal amount of heat, but lose less than the normal amount
of heat, our temperature rises. Speaking generally, the increase of temperature is usually due to our not losing the

G

normal amount by evaporation. This brings us to the more practical part of our subject. As heat materially assists in producing rapid evaporation, the application of it is frequently employed for this purpose, and the temperature is thus lowered.

Heat can be either dry or moist. We can bear the application of dry heat at a much higher temperature than that of moist heat. An excess of dry heat *burns;* an excess of moist heat *scalds.* The temperature of dry heat which can comfortably be tolerated, in a Turkish bath, for instance, would scald if it were moist heat. The atmosphere can only absorb a certain amount of moisture. If the atmosphere has absorbed its full amount evaporation cannot take place, and one chief means of losing heat is prevented.

Heat, both moist and dry, can be subdivided in the same way as we have treated rest and cold—in the general application of it to the whole body, and the partial application of it to relieve or cure locally. To-night we will consider the *general* application of heat, both dry and moist. The effect of dry heat, applied generally, is to produce perspiration, and that is the object for which it is ordered, as a hot air bath, for instance. The object and effect of dry heat when applied partially is to impart heat to the part with which it is placed in contact, as in a hot bottle or brick. General *moist* heat is prescribed with a view to its sedative effect, and this is the remedial property for which it is ordered in conditions both of nervous and muscular excitement, as after great fatigue, etc.

Now we will proceed to the details of the application of general heat both dry and moist. Hot packing is sometimes employed in cases of dropsy, uræmia, etc. The patient's body linen should be removed, and a mackintosh placed over the mattress, covered with a warm dry blanket. Hot packs are ordered at a varying temperature, usually 100° Fahrenheit when no special directions are given, but it must be remembered that if the patient is to be enveloped in a wet sheet or blanket at the temperature prescribed, the water in which it is steeped must be at the very least 10° higher than that, or the orders will not be accurately carried out. The higher the temperature, up to 100° at any rate, the more comfortable the application is likely to prove to the patient. When the choice rests with you, a wet sheet is much more adapted to the purpose than a wet blanket, the latter being very heavy and cumbersome to arrange, and if the patient is quickly covered up with mackintosh and blankets the heat is effectually retained. Patients are usually kept in a hot pack for about an hour, but they may remain longer if comfortable, Occasionally it has a soothing effect, and induces sleep. In taking a patient out of a hot pack it is best to remove the mackintoshes and everything that has become saturated with moisture, and leave him rolled up for a short time in a warm dry blanket. This has a tendency to increase the action of the skin, and lessens the risk of chill. Finally the patient should be comfortably dried with warm towels, great care being taken for some time after the pack that he is not exposed to any draughts, and that all chances of cold, such as an open window during the process of being put comfortable and having the bed made be observantly and scrupulously guarded against.

Hot air baths are frequently ordered for dropsy cases. A long cradle, or sometimes more than one, if you have not one of sufficient length, must be placed in the bed, and the hot air apparatus fitted in at or near the foot. The sheets and the patient's night dress must be removed, and it is well to put a mackintosh beneath the blanket on which the patient is to lie to ensure the bed or mattress being kept quite dry and clean. The blanket placed over the cradle must be carefully tucked under the patient's chin and round the edges of the bed, the blanket covering the patient during the arrangement of the bed being now removed and placed over, not under, the cradle, the whole being finally covered with a mackintosh, and arranged in such a way as to prevent the escape of the hot air.

Miss Florence Lees gives the usual temperature as varying from 100° to 160° Fahr., and the usual duration of the hot air or lamp bath as twenty minutes, but both time and temperature vary according to the cases and the views of the physicians who prescribe them, and you must, of course, endeavour to carry out the orders given in each case.

After the lamp has been removed, the patient should be allowed to perspire freely and to cool a little before being thoroughly dried with a warm towel. A warm night dress should then be put on, and the moist blankets replaced with dry, warm bedding.

A warm bath or a vapour bath prior to a hot air bath increases the effect. Sponging with warm water whilst in the bath is sometimes ordered with a view to increasing the action of the skin. Baths both for medical and cleansing purposes, depend for their successful application upon the efficiency of the nurse. Ordinary cleansing baths are usually given at a temperature of not more than 80° to 92° Fahr. Of course a patient must not be allowed to have a bath until you have asked the sister, but when there is no reason to the contrary, a bath is a quicker and more effectual method of making a patient clean and comfortable than the slower process of washing them all over, as you are frequently obliged to do.

Never leave a patient alone in a bath if you are responsible for it. No doubt you have all heard of accidents at children's and other hospitals occurring from neglect of this rule. In warm baths some patients with weak hearts or in a weak state of health are apt to faint, and some are quickly depressed in cold baths, so that, however sure you may feel that no contingency of the sort is likely to arise, you have no right to run the risk.

The temperature of baths varies somewhat as follows: tepid baths, 85° to 92° Fahr.; warm baths, 92° to 98° Fahr.; hot baths, 98° to 105° Fahr.; 112° Fahr. would be very hot. A hot bath ranges from the temperature of the body upwards; vapour baths, 122° to 144° Fahr. The scale of temperature varies slightly at different places, but I believe this is about the usual average. I give you these particulars for general guidance when you do not receive precise directions, but whenever you are in doubt about what is best for any case in the wards always ask the sister.

Let me strongly recommend you to get into the habit of using the bath thermometer on all occasions. Experience will give you a tolerably correct idea of about what temperature the water is, but not unless you have employed the thermometer regularly, and thus learnt exactly what water feels like at the varying temperatures recorded. In using the thermometer remember that it must be thoroughly immersed in the water for a few seconds before reading it, and not a little water scooped up just to cover the bulb, as I have known some nurses consider sufficient, or of course it will not give the true temperature of the full quantity of water. It is always best for a nurse to be strictly accurate over every detail in which it is in her power to be so, instead of having to report vaguely that it is "about so and so."

When a patient is ordered a bath for medicinal purposes, at a certain temperature, you are intended to *keep* the bath as nearly as possible at that temperature all the time the patient is using it. If you content yourself with giving it to the patient at the required temperature to begin with, it is evident that you will not be carrying out your orders efficiently. To do this you must have a supply of hot water

at hand to add from time to time, and take care to pour it
in gently and slowly *by the side of the bath,* so that the patient
may not fear being scalded.

See that you have everything quite ready before disturbing the patient, so that he or she may not have the fatigue
of waiting about, and the risk of getting a chill. In this as
in other things of the sort, a nurse who has a head and uses
it will save both her patient and herself a great deal of time
and trouble.

As a hot bath induces perspiration patients should have
a blanket wrapped round them, and not be allowed to stay in
a draught or near an open window, neither should they be
allowed to walk about the ward on any pretext whatever
until the immediate effect of the bath upon the skin has
passed off. Unless specially ordered, a patient should not
remain in a hot bath longer than eight or ten minutes.

Hip baths are useful when it is considered desirable to
immerse that part of the body only. When it is a hot hip
bath ordered for medicinal purposes, an even temperature
should be maintained, and a blanket thrown over the patient.
People who have a feeble circulation are sometimes ordered
to take a cold hip bath and a warm foot bath at the same
time, as I said just now.

Arm and leg baths are much used now for surgical cases.
You must take care to place them and the patients in such
a position that they may be as little fatigued and uncomfortable as possible. It is a tiring remedy for patients, owing to
the length of time they are sometimes required to keep the
limb immersed. In this case also the nurse must maintain
the temperature ordered.

Mercurial vapour baths are contrived in various ways,
and the best methods must be learnt by practical observation.

Mustard baths are frequently ordered. The mustard
must be put in a bag or tied up in a piece of flannel or linen

after the fashion of a blue bag. The quantity of mustard varies according to circumstances.

Sulphur and tar baths are sometimes ordered, but for these you will receive special directions in each case.

The application of moist heat mitigates or removes the pain of colic; it relieves spasms; it takes down inflammation. Immersion in very hot water is said to relieve sprains. Hot water applied to the feet and legs sometimes removes headache. Sponging with very hot water will occasionally relieve severe headache when cold treatment altogether fails. The prolonged application of hot baths or any form of heat is said to be weakening.

In our next lecture we will consider this subject further, and more particularly with reference to the local applications of heat as applied in the form of poultices, fomentations, and other remedies of a similar kind.

LECTURE V.

WE have now to consider the details of the various forms in which heat can be applied locally as a remedial agent. We completed the subject of the general application of heat, both dry and moist, at our last lecture, and the partial application of heat can be conveniently subdivided under the same headings.

I should· remind you, to begin with, that the effect of dry heat applied generally is to produce perspiration, and that is the object for which it is ordered, as, for example, a hot air bath.

The object of dry heat, when applied partially, is to impart heat to that portion of the body with which it is placed in contact. The partial application of moist heat is ordered with a view of softening the skin, and thus relieving tension and pain. The early application of moist heat has a tendency to cut short inflammation, as you may sometimes have noticed when a poultice has been applied to a bad finger directly it becomes painful. The effect of a poultice when applied later is to encourage discharge, and so to favour healing.

Dry heat, as I told you last time, can be tolerated at a much higher temperature than moist. Dry heat for local application is usually ordered in the form of hot bottles, bricks, bags filled with hot salt, bran, camomile leaves, or other herbs, to impart heat to the place in question, and to relieve pain. The latter are not often employed in hospital practice, but the application of hot water bottles or tins is very familiar to you, as they are in daily use both in medical and surgical wards.

Of all the times when the hot water tins should be refilled as a matter of daily routine, the early morning is, perhaps, the most important, and I am afraid that this is the time when many nurses and probationers are careless about attending to them. The vital powers of the patients are at their lowest, and nearly all your bad cases are worse than in the evening, when they are more inclined to be warm and comfortable. It is bad management for a nurse to think that the fact of her being busy excuses or explains why her patients should be cold.

When you have a large ward full of patients on your hands, it is not to be expected that you can stay to fill every hot bottle, when perhaps you have a dozen beds to make in a very short space of time; indeed, it would be bad management to do so. The right plan is for night nurses and probationers to refill hot water bottles in the very early morning; then, when day nurses and probationers come on duty and make the beds, the bottle serves as a sensible footstool for such patients as may only just be able to move from their beds while they are made, and there will be no need for the foot warmers to be attended to again until the wards are all straight, and there is leisure to see after them. Moreover, the patients will have had the benefit of them exactly when they were most needed, instead of having to wait until " nurse has time."

Whilst I am speaking of hot water bottles, there are one or two points in connection with them that I may as well mention to you. Always take care that a sheet, blanket, or some covering is placed between the patient and the surface of the hot water bottle or tin. The contact with it makes the skin tender, and is often startling and uncomfortable to the patient if he is awake, and will rouse him suddenly if he happens to be asleep. Do not be satisfied with yourselves until you can take the hot water bottle or tin out of and put it in the bed without waking your patient.

I think you cannot be told too soon of the special risk there is of raising scalds and blisters on paralyzed and dropsy cases, especially the former, by bottles that would not be hot enough to affect other cases in the same way. I hope you will remember this, because you may any day be told to place plenty of hot water bottles in the bed with these patients, and it would be distressing for you to find that through ignorance of this peculiarity you had inadvertently hurt the patient in this way. He might not be conscious of the pain, or not able to call your attention to it; but any wounds in these cases are very slow to heal, and it is necessary to take extreme care to avoid them.

I do not think there are any special points to which I need call your attention in connection with the other methods in which dry heat is sometimes applied.

Moist heat is usually prescribed locally in the form of fomentations and poultices of various kinds. Fomentations are preferable to poultices on the ground that they are cleaner of application, easier made, and easier borne by the patient, but the drawback is that they do not retain the heat nearly so long. The best material to use for fomentation is coarse flannel or soft old blankets.

A wringer, made like a small roller towel, should be placed over a bowl, with the two sticks ready in each side of it, and the flannel placed ready for quite boiling water to be poured on it. It must then be wrung out as dry as it is possible to make it, by turning the sticks rapidly in opposite directions and keeping them as far apart as the size of the wringer will permit. Then untwist and slip out the sticks as quickly as possible, give the fomentation flannel a good shake, and place it lightly on the patient, covering it up with mackintosh or other waterproof material, which is placed over the fomentation with the twofold object of retaining the heat and keeping the patient dry. Nothing is so excellent for this purpose as spongio-piline. The soft side absorbs the moisture from the flannel, and the waterproof side keeps the damp from coming through. To render it quite effectual, the edges should be bevelled inwards, so that the waterproof portion completely covers the whole. This should be placed before the fire to keep it warm, ready for use, while the fomentation is being prepared. Fomentations to be effectual should be changed every ten minutes or quarter of an hour, and I am sure any one who has ever experienced the relief they give in severe pain will be of this opinion. Another flannel should always be wrung out ready to replace the cool one, that the patient may not be kept waiting while the same flannel is made hot. The cool flannel and the wringer should be hung up to dry in readiness for the next application. This appears a trifling detail to which to call your attention, but experience shows that in some cases it is essential to mention it. Fomentations are uncomfortable, and of no service if allowed to remain on too long without changing.

Sometimes fomentation flannels are ordered to be wrung out of a decoction of poppy heads, or other herbs, instead of boiling water. In this case they do not require changing quite so frequently. To make this poppy water, Miss Florence Lees give the following receipt: Take four ounces of dried poppy heads, break them to pieces, and empty out the seeds; then boil the *shells* in three pints of water for a quarter of an hour; strain and keep the water for use.

Mallow water and camomile flower water are made in the

same way, and frequently camomile blossoms are boiled with
the poppy heads.   Sometimes a few drops of laudanum or
tincture of belladonna, or ether, or chloroform, are ordered to
be sprinkled upon the fomentation flannel after it is wrung
out, for the purpose of relieving pain.   Turpentine is occasionally ordered to be sprinkled on the flannel.   This is
usually spoken of as a turpentine stoup.

Miss Wood recommends from thirty to sixty drops of
turpentine ; Miss Lees from one to two tablespoonfuls, which
I consider excessive, unless the turpentine is mixed with the
boiling water before the flannel is wrung out ; but, as the
turpentine floats on the top of the water, unless it is used
instantly, this is not very generally done, nor a desirable
method.   Unless you have distinct orders as to quantity, you
must use your own judgment, and remember turpentine is a
powerful irritant, and that it is necessary for you to be both
careful in the application and watchful in the use of it,
especially with old people and children.   It will break the
skin very quickly if you are careless about it, and we have
already agreed that the aim of skilful nursing is to carry out
orders efficiently, without causing one moment's *unnecessary*
pain or discomfort.   Spongio-piline or a double layer of lint
will form a good substitute for flannel when the latter cannot
be had, but coarse white flannel is generally considered the
best and most comfortable material for the purpose when it
can be obtained, covered with spongio-piline if possible
instead of mackintosh.

When you are briefly told to apply a poultice, and no
further particulars are given, you will take it for granted
that it is to be made of linseed-meal, and in hospitals this is
generally made on tow instead of linen.

To make a linseed-meal poultice properly, you require a
poultice bowl, a basin, a poultice spatula, a poultice board,
and a little olive oil, in addition, of course, to boiling water,

linseed-meal, and the tow or linen. Pour a little boiling water into the poultice bowl, and place the blade of the spatula in it, while you prepare the tow. A verbal description of how to prepare the tow will scarcely give you a very clear idea of it, but any day you can have a practical illustration of this in the wards, the object, of course, being to make it smooth and of an even thickness. Then pour the water, which has been warming the poultice bowl ready for your use, into the basin, and pour boiling water sufficient to make the size poultice you require into the warmed poultice bowl. Only observation and experience can teach you to judge of the quantity, but this you will soon learn. Then take linseed-meal in your left hand, and sprinkle it freely into the water, rapidly stirring with the right hand in one direction all the while. It should be made of the consistency of porridge, just thick enough to be cleanly cut with the spatula. It must then be rapidly spread on the tow, and the spatula should be frequently dipped into the basin of hot water, partly to prevent the poultice sticking to the spatula, and also to make it spread smoothly.

Different opinions prevail as to the thickness of a linseed-meal poultice. Miss Wood says, in her "Handbook of Nursing," that it should be "about one-eighth to a quarter of an inch thick," which I consider too thin. Dr. Smith, in his excellent "Lectures on Nursing," says "half an inch thick," as the general rule, and that is the advice I recommend you to follow. You must endeavour to avoid the two extremes of making the poultice too thick and heavy, which is very objectionable, and of making it too thin, so that it does not retain the heat.

You must leave a border of tow, or of linen, if you are making it on that material, all round, which must be lightly rolled back upon the poultice, and a little olive oil may be sprinkled and smoothed over it to prevent sticking,

and to cool the surface. Even without the oil, if the poultice
has been properly made, and the spatula dipped in hot water
passed lightly over it, it should never stick, either to the
patient or to itself when folded together. A nurse will always
know that her poultice falls short of perfection if it adheres
to the skin in the least. For children it is always best to use
a little oil, because the cool surface enables them to bear the
poultice applied warmer than they will do otherwise.

Poultices should be put on as warm as the patient can
comfortably bear them, unless contrary orders are given; but
great care must be taken not to scald, and it must also be
remembered that frequent applications to the same place make
it tender, so that it is probable for this reason that the patient
may not be able to bear repeated poultices quite as warm as
the first. Always *make* them as hot as possible, for they cool
rapidly, and a poultice put on cooler than it could comfortably
have been borne is not satisfactory. Never put a poultice in
the oven to keep hot; it only dries and hardens it, rendering
it quite unfit for use. If it happens that you are obliged to
keep it waiting before using it, place it between two hot
plates over a saucepan or kettle of boiling water, but never
do this when it can be avoided.

Always prepare your patient as much as possible before
making your poultice, but without removing the former
poultice until you have the fresh one there ready to put on.
In surgical cases, where the wound requires washing, that
should be attended to, the poultice removed, and the part
covered with wet lint to keep the air from it while the fresh
poultice is made; but I am speaking more particularly of
medical poultices now, and not so much of those which come
under the head of dressings.

For instance, in bad chest cases, where perhaps you have
a large jacket poultice made in two parts and bound on with
a rib bandage, take the precaution to unwind the bandage,

and have that or another one wound ready for use before you begin to make the poultice, taking care to replace the poultice, covering one-half before removing the other part, and thus avoiding the risk of chill. When you have learnt to be very quick, and your patient is not too exhausted to bear it, it is a good plan to wipe over the place where the poultice has been applied very gently and rapidly with a small piece of lint or cotton wool, because the air coming to the moist surface gives it an uncomfortable itching sensation; but do not let your patient and the poultice get cold together while you are interesting yourself with picking off any little dry bits that may have adhered to the patient.

For medical cases, where there is no wound, you must put a piece of thin mackintosh or other waterproof material over the poultice, because it will keep it moist and warm for a much longer period, and thus save the patient the fatigue of having it changed so often. Gutta percha tissue is not a good material for this purpose, although it is waterproof, because it shrivels up with the heat and smells objectionable. Poultices applied in this manner usually require changing every four hours, and would need to be renewed oftener but for the covering.

Large poultices keep warm for a much longer period than small ones, so that in making small poultices you must be particular that everything you use is thoroughly warmed, and they will need to be renewed more frequently. It is a good plan to change large poultices every four hours, and small poultices every two hours, when no orders are given. Of course, when orders *are* given, you have only to carry them out, whatever they may be.

Poultices applied to wounds must not be covered up with mackintosh, and all surgical poultices must be very light, and the size carefully adapted to the requirements of the case. If they are ordered for the purpose of bringing forward an abscess, they should be as warm as the patient can comfortably bear them, and frequently renewed.

A few drops of laudanum sprinkled on the surface of the poultice is often very effectual for soothing pain, but be especially careful if ever you are ordered to use this for children, and never exceed the quantity prescribed. It may be as well to take this opportunity of reminding you that children are peculiarly susceptible to the influence of this drug, and can never bear its application in any form in anything approaching to the same proportion as adults.

Sometimes linseed-meal poultices are made with a decoction of poppy heads or other herbs instead of boiling water, and that often affords relief in severe pain. Linseed-meal poultices are always placed next the skin, and should never have a covering of muslin, nor anything else between.

In applying poultices to paralyzed or dropsy cases the same warning which I gave you in reference to hot water bottles must be remembered. I mean the extreme liability of these cases to become scalded on the application of any hot substance at a temperature not sufficiently high to produce a similar result in other conditions of the body.

Charcoal poultices are frequently ordered for a wound where there is a great deal of fœtid discharge. The simplest method of making them is to mix one part of charcoal with two parts of linseed-meal, and then make the poultice in the ordinary way. This is cleaner and more effectual than sprinkling the charcoal on the surface of the linseed-meal poultice, as is sometimes done. The same purpose is served in a much cleaner and nicer way by mixing linseed-meal with boiling coal-tar lotion instead of water.

Some skill and practice is required to make a good bread poultice, for it is apt to become either heavy, lumpy, and sloppy, or dry, hard, and sticky. The best method of preparing them is first to get ready a sufficient supply of

bread crumbs, and then stir them into the boiling water
exactly in the same way as you would linseed-meal, stirring
and beating it rapidly all the while. Then cover it up with
a plate or saucer, and leave it by the fire, or, better still, over
a kettle of boiling water for about five minutes to give it time
to swell. Then spread it on linen—never on tow—dipping
the spatula into hot water to prevent sticking, and turn up
the outside margin of linen in the usual way. You will
need some olive oil or simple dressing to spread on the
surface—the latter *looks* best, but either will do—because
bread has a great tendency to stick, and it hurts very much
if dry, hard, little pieces have to be picked off the edges of a
wound.

You cannot roll bread poultices up in the same way
that you can linseed-meal, nor fold them up to take to a
patient, or they will break and fall to pieces. They are
applied either hot or cold, according to orders. It will
save time and trouble if you make a sufficient supply at
one time for two or three poultices, as the preparation does
not spoil, unless it is left long enough to turn sour, and it
can easily be warmed afresh over a kettle of boiling water, or
by the addition of a little hot water to the soaked bread.
Bread poultices are placed next the skin.

Mustard and linseed-meal poultices are frequently used.
The difficulty of mixing these ingredients is obviated here
by your having the material prepared from the dispensary.
When you have to prepare this poultice for yourselves,
the best method is to put the mustard first into the boiling
water, and see that it is thoroughly mixed before adding the
linseed-meal in the usual way. By this means you avoid the
risk of the mustard remaining in patches to irritate the
skin.

But in recommending this plan I must be careful to explain to you that the mustard can only be mixed with boiling

H

water when the object is to secure a diffused redness over the whole surface to which the linseed-meal poultice has been applied, and not when it is desired to produce the maximum irritating effect for which mustard plasters are prescribed. A lesser and sufficient irritation is effectually produced in the manner described, and the discomfort of the mustard stinging in little patches avoided. The reason why mustard should not be mixed with boiling water under other circumstances was clearly explained to me by an eminent physician in a kindly criticism on my " Lecture on Home Nursing," where I briefly gave the suggestion referred to for making a mustard and linseed-meal poultice. He said, " The value of mustard as an external application is due to volatile oil, which does not pre-exist in the mustard, but is produced by the action, when moistened, of a body called myrosine on another body called myronic acid. The myrosine acts like a ferment on the myronic acid, and *produces* the oil. Hot water, and especially boiling water, coagulates the myrosine, prevents its action on the myronic acid, and fails in *producing* the oil, or at any rate diminishes its formation." It is therefore not difficult to understand why mustard must never be mixed with boiling water when its maximum effect is desired.

If these poultices are ordered for a continuance, and the skin appears likely to break in places, you must cover these spots with very small pieces of lint or linen, spread with zinc ointment or simple dressing, before applying the poultice, and then the patient will not be obliged to discontinue remedies which may be deemed necessary for his case in consequence of the local discomfort.

Mustard-leaves that you procure from a chemist are nearly always used now in preference to plasters, but they are a great deal more painful. When you have mustard plasters to prepare, they are made with mustard mixed to a paste with cold or tepid water. A little flour may be added, but not necessarily so. It is sometimes desirable to precede a mustard plaster with a linseed-meal poultice, or to bathe the part to which it is applied with very hot water, in order to make the mustard plaster produce its maximum effect.

Some people and books tell us that mustard plasters are best made on brown paper, covered with brown paper or muslin. I prefer tissue paper entirely. Several folds of tissue paper make a sufficiently thick and satisfactory background for spreading the mustard on, and one piece folded over the surface can be neatly doubled back over the edges. Tissue paper is better than muslin, as the mustard cannot so readily get through; mustard plasters are *not* placed next to the skin, and must not be made too wet. They should be fastened on with two or three pieces of strapping to keep them in place, and covered with a little cotton wool to absorb any moisture, and prevent any soiling of such clothes as may come in contact with it. Do not allow the plaster to remain on long enough to break the skin or raise a blister, and be specially careful in this respect with children and old people. With these cases it is best to remove the mustard plaster rather quickly, and replace it by a linseed-meal poultice for a time, which will render the mustard application effectual without the risk of a troublesome sore. As a rule, have a piece of linen spread with simple dressing or zinc ointment ready to put on when you remove the plaster, as it relieves the burning, tingling sensation, and then replace the cotton wool over it.

There are several other kinds of poultices, such as carrot, yeast, chlorinated soda, and so on; but these are ordered comparatively seldom, and it is best for you to have directions from the doctor who prescribes them of the exact way in which he wishes them made, as I am anxious for you, in the first instance, to learn those things which it is absolutely

essential you should know.   In this, as in other details, I am
endeavouring to explain to you what experience proves to be
the best method to take for a general rule, but I do this
always with the understanding that in practical work you
obey the instructions of those under whom you may be
immediately working for the time being.

LECTURE VI.

WE have, for the present, finished our consideration of the application of cold and heat as remedial agents. The last detail that we spoke of was a mustard plaster, and we may fairly consider that this leads us to the question of counter-irritation. Under this head I should like to bring to your notice especially the process of dry and wet cupping, leeches, and blisters.

But, first of all, what do we understand by counter-irritation? We mean the application of an irritant sufficient even to produce inflammation to the surface, to counteract a deeper-seated inflammation. Fortunately, it does not rest with us to inquire in what manner this result is brought about. We have only to deal with the plain fact that, some-how or other, counter-irritation does produce this effect.

There are different degrees of counter-irritation; first, a mere increase of vascularity, i.e., the drawing of an increased supply of blood to the surface, which I told you was one of the results of a hot application, and as the normal amount of blood in the body remains to all intents and purposes same in ordinary circumstances, the drawing of this additional supply of blood to the surface implies the withdrawing of it from some interior organs. Now this object may be attained to some extent by the application of poultices and fomenta-tions only, or aided by the addition of turpentine, etc., to these. The same object can be attained to a greater extent by dry cupping, and to a still greater extent by wet cupping and leeches, as that involves the withdrawal of a certain amount of blood, not only *to* the surface, but *from* the body altogether.

The second degree of counter-irritation may be an increase of vascularity, combined with a certain amount of inflammation, such as is best illustrated, perhaps, by a mustard plaster, which, as you know, not only increases the vascularity of the part to which it is applied, but sets up a certain amount of inflammation of the surface at the same time.

The third degree of counter-irritation produces true inflammation, amounting to a blister, and we will endeavour to speak of all these in detail to-night.

First, then, let us turn our attention to the means of applying the first degree of counter-irritation, the object of which is to create a mere increase of vascularity, *i.e.*, the drawing of an increased supply of blood to the surface. The simplest method of attaining this object is by poultices and fomentations; but we have already minutely considered the preparation and application of these. We will now proceed to the study of cupping and leeches.

Cupping is of two kinds—dry and wet. It is resorted to somewhat less frequently now, for the most part, than it was in former times, and it is not very often done by the nurse. Still you should be competent to do it, if you receive orders to that effect. There are glasses of various sizes made for the purpose, which I dare say some of you have seen or will see in the wards. In addition to these are required a spirit lamp, spirits of wine, blotting paper, cotton wool, a saucer for wet cupping, and a scarificator.

The glasses are warmed, and should then have the air exhausted from them by inserting pieces of wool or blotting-paper dipped in the spirit, and setting them on fire in the glass itself. Your finger should be dipped in oil and passed rapidly round the edge of the glass before it is applied.

After that the glass should be placed quickly on the selected spot, and gently pressed on it, so that the edges may fit closely to the surface, care being taken not to heat the glass too much, lest the patient should be scorched.   The skin will then rise within the glass, which can easily be removed when desired by inserting the nail of the thumb under the edge of the glass and pressing the skin downwards. This is *dry* cupping, and is generally employed to relieve pain.

Wet cupping is performed in a similar manner except that the glass is removed, and a scarificator immediately applied to the part, and then the glass at once re-applied as before.   The hemorrhage can be readily stopped, when desired, by a pad of dry lint.   The usual site for wet-cupping is the loins, just over the kidneys, and it is generally used for inflammation of those organs, but it is also of service in relieving pain in other regions.

Leeches are used for the purpose of taking away a small quantity of blood, and they must never be applied over any large vessel.   Sometimes it is difficult to get them to bite at all, or to make them fasten on the desired spot.   The part should be washed perfectly clean with soap and water, and that is often sufficient preparation.   If they will not take, the part should be moistened with a little milk, or sugar and water, or a little prick or scratch be made, so that a drop of blood will exude upon the surface.

The less the leeches are handled the better as a rule, but unless they are applied in water they are best wiped dry with a soft towel.   Miss Wood recommends that they should be kept out of water for a short time before they are used, and considers that this renders them more inclined to bite.   Dr. Smith and Miss Lees, on the contrary, recommend their application in water for the reason that water is their native element, and that when they are cool and comfortable in it they will settle at once.   If they are very tiresome you can

put them in a wine glass full of water, cover it with a piece
of paper, and turn it upside down on the place where you
wish the leech to settle, putting a towel underneath to soak
up the water then, and when the leech has taken, you
remove the glass altogether. It is not, however, necessary to
do this unless the leeches decline to bite in the ordinary way.

If you want to apply a leech close to the eye, or have had
particular orders as to the exact spot upon which it is
desired to fasten, fill a test tube with water and put a leech
in it, or stuff the tube half full of cotton wool and then put
the leech in. If you put them into this small compass you
must see that their heads and not their tails are at the mouth
of the tube, otherwise, as they have not room to turn round,
there will be no possibility of their fulfilling their mission.

Dr. Stoke says, " Take half an apple, scrape out the pulp,
and, placing the leeches in, invert the rind on to the skin.
Leeches thus applied will bite at once."

I have never tried this plan nor seen it tried, but one can
readily conceive it to be excellent, as containing the leeches
in a small compass, and as being a soft, light material to
place against the patient; whereas the rim of a wine-glass
might press rather heavily if it were not gently used.

When the leeches have once fastened to the required spot
they must be left undisturbed. When they have finished
they generally drop off, but if any of them should remain
sticking an unusually long time, they must never be forcibly
pulled away, or the teeth may be left in the wound. If it is
necessary to do anything, a little salt sprinkled on them will
cause them speedily to relinquish their hold.

Each leech is said to obtain rather less than one drachm
or teaspoonful, but warm fomentations will materially increase
this quantity if desired. If, on the other hand, there is any
difficulty in arresting the bleeding, the pressure of the finger,
a little dry linseed-meal sprinkled on the surface, a small pad

of cotton wool or dry lint, a cold compress, or a little ice—
any one of these things will probably be sufficient to stop it.
If the bleeding persists after trying these remedies, a little
tincture of iron diluted, or a point of caustic inserted into
the leech bites is generally effectual, but you would not apply
these without orders from the doctor, unless you were nursing
a case in which it was not possible to obtain his assistance.

In most cases, where no special orders are given, when
the leeches are removed, just wipe over the wounds with
a bit of cotton wool, and leave a piece over the place. It will
absorb any slight bleeding that occurs, and is comfortable for
the patient. The nurse must see occasionally that no bleeding
is going on, for it may do so to a considerable extent before
the patient is aware of it. The night nurse should also watch
for bleeding after leeches, not that it is likely to occur, but
cases have happened where serious harm has been done from
the bites bleeding profusely during the patient's sleep.
Some persons have a peculiar tendency to bleed freely, and it
is well that you should be aware of this, in case you should
meet with any instances of it.

Some nurses and some patients have a particular dislike
to leeches, and feel quite afraid of them, while others, on the
contrary, do not mind them at all. Nurses who have this
dislike must endeavour not to show it, for the sake of the
patients, and be careful not to make them nervous ; and nurses
who have no personal objection to leeches must not be unmindful of the feelings of those who have, and avoid teasing
them, for I am inclined to believe that the sort of unreasonable horror which some people have of these harmless little
creatures is by no means nonsense or affectation, but a kind
of innate aversion to them which cannot easily be overcome.

After the leeches have been used they should be put
with a little salt, which will cause them to vomit the blood,
and they can then be placed in fresh cold water, which will

require changing occasionally if they are to be kept in the ward.

The second degree of counter-irritation may be an increase of vascularity combined with a certain amount of irritation, such as is illustrated by a mustard-plaster, which, as you already know, not only increases the vascularity of the part to which it is applied, but renders it very sensitive, and sets up a certain amount of inflammation of the surface.

The third degree of counter-irritation produces true inflammation, amounting to a blister. Blisters may, of course, be produced by the careless administration of almost any of these hot applications; but even if an accident of the sort is not attended with any special harm to the patient, that fortunate circumstance does not exonerate a nurse from blame if she has produced a blister by the way she has applied an agent that was only intended to act as a counter-irritant in a minor degree, or perhaps not designed to procure that effect at all, for poultices and fomentations are more frequently ordered for other purposes, and stronger measures are used when counter-irritation is desired.

Blisters, as such, are produced by the ordinary blister plaster, or by painting with a blistering fluid. The latter is the least uncomfortable, for when the fluid begins to accumulate underneath the cuticle, the sticking of the plaster on the skin round the surface where the blister is placed greatly increases the discomfort. For this reason it is best not to apply blisters with strapping, or at any rate with only one piece to keep it in place, and cover it with some cotton wool. If the blister has been applied on a plaster it must be removed very gently when the cuticle has risen, for the part will have become extremely tender. Before painting with the blistering fluid it is a good plan to define the extent of surface which you intend the blister to cover with a slight outline of olive oil. This, with a little care, has the happy effect of preventing the blistering fluid from spreading beyond the desired spot. Probationers have often to learn at the cost of some discomfort to the patient that if a little of the fluid runs down by the side of the place to which the blister is being applied, wiping it rapidly does not prevent the irritation extending to every spot with which the fluid has come in contact. It is especially useful to employ the oil and prevent any accident of the kind in nursing children.

There are cases in which the oily matter of the skin prevents the blister from rising. This difficulty in the rare instances in which it occurs can be overcome by wiping the place to which the blister is to be applied with a little ether. The time a blister takes to rise varies in different people and in different parts of the body, from six to twelve hours, but the nurse should watch its progress from time to time. Sometimes the blister is very slow to rise, and then a warm poultice should be applied over it, which will materially aid the process. The exact spot and extent of the blister should be definitely ordered by the doctor, but sometimes the order is given so vaguely that a nurse is rather puzzled what to do. Of course in the wards you can always ask the sister, but for those who are private nursing, for instance, it may be useful to know that, as a rule, blisters applied to joints are more effectual if placed in the region of the joint and not immediately over it. Thus, a blister for the hip-joint is most effectual if applied in the region of the groin ; for the knee-joint if applied in the shape of two half-moons above and below the knee-cap ; for the ankle if put between that joint and the heel, and so on. To dress the blister, place a small receiver, or, if the blister is very small, a towel or a piece of lint or wool close underneath to receive the fluid, and then make a snip at the most depending part of the vesicle. Press very gently over the raised cuticle, and see that all the serum comes out. After which, apply the dressing—usually simple

dressing, olive oil, or zinc ointment on linen or lint over the
inflamed surface *without removing the cuticle*; be sure you
have it ready, and not keep the patient waiting while you
go off to get it; the part will generally heal rapidly. It
must be kept clean, and the dressing renewed twice or more
if necessary, in the twenty-four hours. If it is desired to
keep the blister " open," which is not very often the case,
remove the raised cuticle with a pair of scissors and dress
the place with the irritant application ordered, but be careful
that this is the *exact size of the sore*. A piece of lint spread
with simple dressing or oil a little larger than the sore, should
be placed over the other application, and strapped on to keep
it in place. The wound must be kept clean, and the dressing
re-applied daily until further orders.

I think that is all that I have to bring to your notice in
connection with a nurse's duties when counter-irritation is
the treatment prescribed.

The next detail of nursing to which I am desirous of
calling your attention is one which has to be kept in such
constant remembrance by the nurse, that I can hardly avoid
mentioning it in connection with the special nursing of every
case, and so, to spare you repetition, we will consider this
matter separately—I mean the risk, prevention, and cure of
bed-sores. They are the terror of all good nurses, as most of
you know, and with sufficient reason, for, in the first place,
they are the source of the greatest distress, pain, and discomfort to the unfortunate patient; and, in the second place, in
nine cases out of ten they are the result of carelessness and
neglect, or at any rate they occur from the want of sufficient
care on the part of the nurse. There *are* cases in which no
amount of care can prevent them, but these are comparatively
exceptional, and it is well for all nurses to consider them so.
Doubtless you will have a useful and interesting lecture on
this subject later on, therefore I shall not take it very fully,

but as I feel it is impossible to speak of the trained nursing of operation, accident, and many medical cases, without dwelling upon this important item, I cannot pass it over here altogether.

Bed-sores are the result of pressure, as you all know, therefore a nurse's object is to relieve pressure on all the more prominent and sensitive parts. The lower part of the back and the hip bones are the parts needing most care and watching as a rule, but in certain conditions bed-sores will also occur on the heels, elbows, knees, ankles, if these joints are in such a position as to come in close contact with the bed or pillows. The next thing to be avoided is moisture, for that is the second condition that will speedily induce bed-sores unless it is very carefully guarded against; and moisture, when combined with pressure, materially increases the tendency to them.

A nurse's business chiefly lies in the prevention of bed-sores, for in most cases the surgeon prescribes the treatment when the sore has occurred. You all know the necessity for keeping the patient as dry as possible. If this is not done other means are useless. Be very careful but very firm about this point, and use all your ingenuity in difficult cases to attain this all-important object of keeping the patient perfectly dry. Now, in cases where the patient is lying in one position long, you must not wait until some signs of redness appear before you begin taking the necessary precautions. You must guard against the tendency from the very first, as an evil that will inevitably attempt to come, if it does not succeed. It is good to cleanse the parts thoroughly with soap and water, and afterwards powder them freely with zinc powder or starch. Some doctors do not approve of washing with soap and water, and when you have orders to the contrary, you have only to obey, and avoid criticising them; but I am now giving you general rules for your own personal guidance when these matters are left to you.

Spirit is extremely useful, and should be freely rubbed into and allowed to dry into the part *when the skin is not broken.* When it *is* broken, continue to rub the neighbouring parts with spirit, carefully avoiding the sore place. Some nurses forget to continue this when a sore has begun. A very effectual way of applying powder and spirit when you are dealing with a tendency to bed-sore is to moisten a piece of cotton wool with spirit. Dip this into the powder and rub it on. If the skin breaks very little, white of egg is an excellent thing to prevent its getting worse, and it forms a healing sort of glaze over it. Zinc ointment, oil, and spirit, and any greasy application rubbed freely over the parts is excellent where the nature of the case makes it impossible to maintain more than comparative dryness. Of course water rolls off the greasy surface, and neither moistens nor irritates it to the same extent. Never forget the possibility, and in many cases the *probability*, of bed-sore; use all your efforts to prevent it, but remember that the earliest evidence of one must be reported and shown to the doctor. Nothing can excuse any neglect of this rule. The condition of a bed-sore is sometimes an index to the state of a patient's condition in other respects. Some doctors leave the treatment of mild bed-sores in the nurse's hands, some prescribe for it themselves; but take care that you always leave the *responsibility* with them.

Another good plan is to rub a mixture of olive oil and some sort of spirit over the tender part for at least five minutes, two or three times a day. The friction is of great service as well as the ingredients rubbed in.

Collodion painted carefully in one layer over the part is very useful; it excludes the air and allows any slight sore to heal naturally underneath it. But if applying this at night, keep the light at a safe distance, for the ether it contains is extremely inflammable, and I have myself known an instance where the patient was badly burnt from the nurse's careless-ness in reference to, or her ignorance of, this fact.

In some cases a very good result is obtained by dusting the sensitive parts with zinc powder and painting on one layer of flexible collodion over this. This remedy is espe-cially useful in those cases where the constant difficulty is to guard against moisture.

Some surgeons order amadou plaster to be applied with a hole cut in the centre, the size of the sore, to relieve it of all pressure, and when this is ordered of course you will have an opportunity of seeing the effect of it. For the most part I think you will find that this treatment has a tendency to make the surrounding parts tender also. Small circular pillows made with a hole in the centre are most useful for protecting sores where they exist, or the place where they are likely to occur.

The dressing of bed-sores nearly always falls to the nurse's share. Zinc dressing, carbolic oil, resin, iodioform, gall oint-ment, tincture of benzoin, and nitrate of silver are all suitable for varied cases of bed-sores. Water pillows are very desirable for cases where bed-sores are to be anticipated; indeed, paralyzed and dropsy cases should invariably be supplied with them from the first, if possible.

Remember that crumbs in the bed, wrinkles in the bedding and blankets placed under the bottom sheet are all conducive to bed-sores.

I think there is still time for me to say a few words to you in connection with the subject of accidents and emer-gencies—always bearing in mind that these matters will be brought before you much more effectually and in far greater fulness later on.

The first thing you have to consider—supposing the accident beds to be all ready—is the method of undressing the patient so as to avoid unnecessary pain or increasing the extent of the injury. Unskilful handling of a simple fracture will easily turn it into a compound fracture, for instance. Perhaps I should explain, for the benefit of those who are quite new to hospital work, that a fracture is termed simple when the bone is broken and the skin remains un-injured, and compound when the broken bone has pierced the skin.

Cases of fractured femur are perhaps the most difficult to undress. The bedclothes should be turned back to the foot of the bed, and the patient laid in the middle. The coat, waistcoat, and collar should be removed first, as gently and expeditiously as possible. The outside seam of the trousers of the injured leg should then be ripped up, waistband in-cluded—and take care that the buttons of the braces are unfastened at the back as well as the front, to avoid all dragging—then throw a sheet lightly over the patient, to prevent any exposure, and the cut trouser leg must then be drawn, with the utmost care, from under the whole length of the leg to the inside, slipping your hand gently under the thigh, if necessary, to guard against any jerk. You can easily draw off the leg of the trousers of the uninjured side, while the sheet is still over the patient. The stockings must be cut down the seam to the foot, and then taken off without a jerk, by keeping one hand firmly on the ankle. If it is a broken arm, a dislocated shoulder, or any injury of the upper extremity, remove the sleeves from the uninjured side first, *if* it can be done without causing much pain; but if not, the outside seam of coat, waistcoat, and shirt must be ripped up.

Never risk increasing the injury by refraining from cutting the clothes; but the destruction of clothes is a matter of great importance to poor people, and must not be done recklessly. Cut tapes and buttons, bootlaces, and hooks and eyes freely—these can be quickly replaced—but never destroy material when it can judiciously be avoided. Women know

how to undress a woman, but take care and ascertain that
all buttons, strings, etc., are freely unfastened before you
attempt pulling them off. In all cases undress the patient
as though the injury were of a serious nature ; avoid jerks
and pulling. Before taking off the boots, take a firm hold of
the ankle, so that there may be no strain above that. Be
sure and see that the garters are removed before attempting
to draw off the stockings. It seems ridiculous to point out
this, but nurses sometimes forget it. In putting on and
taking off clothing from patients where movement is a
difficulty, lay down for yourselves the distinct rule, "Never
make two separate moves where one would do," and then
reduce this to practice in each case, with all the common
sense that you possess.

Remember, if you are putting on a clean shirt or night-
dress, the bad side must be attended to first ; if you are
taking it off, take out the uninjured side first, so that there
may be no difficulty or strain in getting it off the bad side.

Never touch any wounded limb as though you were afraid
of it ; handle it very gently, of course, but quite firmly. A
hesitating hold will fidget the patient, give unnecessary pain,
and inspire no confidence. While I am speaking of moving
people, I had better remind you that if you have to lift or
carry patients with injuries or diseased limbs, as frequently
happens in the case of children, that the bad side must
always be carried *the furthest away from you*, and the uninjured side next to you. Do not forget this, for you are less
likely to hurt in this manner, and it looks "untrained" to do
it the other way.

If you are putting to bed hip disease cases, for instance,
the patients are frightened at the pain which the least
movement causes them. Let them put their arms round
your neck to support themselves ; or, if it is only a question
of raising themselves in bed, they can do it with the pulley ;

I

and turn all your attention to keeping the limb absolutely
straight. It is best to take a firm hold of the leg above the
ankle, making a little traction at the same time; and, as you
do not want to throw any increased weight on the inflamed
joint of the hip or knee, whichever it may be, keep the head
low and resist the tendency to raise it. When you have the
patient in your arms, remember, if you are assisting in
putting a patient straight and comfortable in bed, and are
asked to raise him, *go on the uninjured side!*

Now, when you have succeeded in undressing your patient,
and he is safely in bed, the next thing is to get him thoroughly
clean, particularly the injured part, as that is what the doctors
will want to deal with first. Patients are generally very
dirty in accident wards. Often they are brought in straight
from work of a dirty nature. Sometimes the shock of the
accident may make it imperative not to disturb the patient
at all, but in that case you must get orders on the subject:
that is the exception, and washing a patient thoroughly as
soon as possible is the rule. You must guard against cold.
The vital powers of the patient will frequently be lowered
from the shock of the accident; be especially careful to keep
this in remembrance with all cases of burns.

All accident beds should be provided with a mackintosh
and draw-sheet to be put on the pillow, near the foot, or in
the middle of the bed, wherever it is needed. If there is no
necessity for it, it can easily be removed, but it should always
be there to begin with. It is useful for the washing process,
if nothing else, and it is dirty, wasteful, and most careless on
the part of a nurse to let the bedding and mattresses get
soaked through with blood before she thinks it necessary to
see after a mackintosh.

Fractures are placed on firm even beds. In some hospitals
fracture-boards are used—*i.e.*, plain deal boards, the size of
the bedsteads—and in other hospitals straw mattresses,

under the hair mattresses, which should be placed over both.
The fracture femur beds in use in the wards will explain
themselves—at least, I need not say anything special about
them here.

Fractures should be placed between sand-bags until further
orders are given. If it is a compound fracture, watch carefully for bleeding, and in these cases have ready a basin of cold
water, sponges, lint, and collodion, in addition to the splints,
pads, bandages, cotton wool, strapping and strapping-tin,
which you would get ready for the surgeon in simple fractures
also. In cases of fractured femur, the patient should lie upon
his back, and only have pillows so as to keep the body as
level as possible. In cases of fractured ribs, the patient will
be more comfortable propped up with pillows, and probably
will prefer to lie on the bad side, as in cases of pleurisy; it
enables him to breathe with less pain. You know the fear
in all cases of fractured ribs is that it may be complicated
with injury to, or inflammation of, the lungs, therefore watch
for any cough or spitting of blood. Do not forget that when
the lower limbs are in splints, and are not slung up in a
cradle, you will have bed-sores on the heels if you do not
guard against them, and take the precautions I have already
mentioned.

In cases of concussion or lacerated scalp, there must be
no shaking, no food must be given, and perfect quiet must
be maintained. You should have ice-bags and hot bottles
quite ready to apply the instant they are ordered. In these
cases notice if there is any discharge from the ears or nose.
There may be squinting, contraction, or dilation of pupils.
Notice also if there is any paralysis, or if any convulsions
occur; if there is involuntary evacuations of the bowels or
bladder, or any vomiting. These things the nurse may be
the first to notice; but remember only to report the occurrence
of any one or more of these symptoms, and do not exceed

your duty by any observation to the effect that they have *not* occurred, except in reply to a direct inquiry from the doctor.

Some of the cases that are carried in to you "insensible" are in this condition from drunkenness. For these patients you should raise the head a little and turn it on one side, for the same reason that you do so for a patient under an anæsthetic—*i.e.*, that is, to avoid the risk of vomited matter being drawn back into the trachea and choking the patient while he is in an unconscious state.

Many of your cases are complicated with *delirium tremens*. I must not linger to describe the symptoms of its coming on at length. Its advent is frequently characterized by bad dreams, temporary wanderings, fussy excitability. Take great care of the injured limb while the patient is in this irresponsible condition.

Fainting comes under the heading of emergencies, if not of accidents. It is caused by the temporary failure of the heart's action, and the consequent cessation of circulation in the brain. Lay the patient flat—to facilitate the flow of blood to the head—and avoid the common mistake of raising the patient. Secure plenty of fresh air, and at the same time guard against cold. Consciousness gradually returns. The distinctions between the insensibility of fainting, of drunkenness, of concusssion and of compression of the brain, cannot fail to be very interesting to you, and will doubtless be pointed out to you in detail by-and-by.

The occurrence of erysipelas is always to be dreaded in accident and surgical wards. It is no part of a nurse's business to diagnose this. Do not say to the doctor, " I think such and such a case has erysipelas because of so and so; " but it is desirable for you to know the symptoms of erysipelas setting in, that you may not fail to notice and report them. Redness round the edges of the wound, vomiting, rigors, the temperature rising, are among the chief. If from what you hear or see you have reason to suppose erysipelas has occurred, it is your duty to take every precaution against carrying the contagion to your other patients. Therefore, *quietly* dip your hands in carbolic acid, and be most scrupulously careful about cleansing and disinfecting any instruments, appliances, or utensils that have been used by or for this case. Do not, for instance, put the bundle of wool, etc., carelessly on the bed whilst doing the dressing, and then carry it off to another bed. If you *can* manage to dress all your other cases first and leave the doubtful one to the last, so much the better. If the case is pronounced erysipelas it will at once be removed from the wards, and then you will only have to be most conscientious in clearing away all bedding, curtains, etc., washing the bedstead with carbolic acid, and taking every precaution that no trace may remain.

I think this is all I have to say to you in connection with this branch of your work.

LECTURE VII.

To-NIGHT I propose to speak, in the first place, of a nurse's duties in connection with operations. We have to consider—the preparation of the patient, the preparation of the theatre, the duties of the nurse in the theatre, the after care of the patient, and then a few details to be remembered for the nursing of special operation cases.

1st. The preparation of the patient.

Many of you know already, and all of you ought to know, the importance of keeping the patient without solid food for at least four or five hours before the administration of ether or chloroform. In many cases beef-tea and brandy is given much later than that, but not solid food, and you must not give anything at all without permission to do so. Some house surgeons give minute directions on this point, and then you have no responsibility beyond carrying them out; but others take it for granted that a nurse is aware of this in- variable rule, and will expect her to attend to it without further reminder, if he merely says that a patient is to be operated upon at a certain hour.

Be sure that you never fail, from any reason whatever, to report the fact if the patient has taken solid food at a later hour than the surgeon is aware; to do so is to risk the patient's life. If you have carelessly forgotten the order that the patient was to be kept without food, let no fear of getting blamed in the matter deter you from reporting the fact *at once;* or if the patient has succeeded in getting food in any other way, you must let the sister know of it immediately. Anæsthetics produce sickness, and the chief risk lies in the vomit being drawn back into the trachea, when the patient is under the influence of ether or chloroform.

An aperient is generally ordered the night before the operation. In operations near the rectum, bladder, or vagina, an enema is nearly always ordered in the morning of the operation. In some hospitals there is a standing rule on this point, but in others special directions are given in each case. In every instance you should give the patients the opportunity of making themselves quite comfortable in these respects the last thing before they are taken to the theatre. When the patients are allowed to have a bath the night before, it is a very desirable thing for them; and if not, you must always see that they are carefully washed.

All dressings must be removed, the wound, if one exists, cleansed, and the place covered with a piece of lint, just before the patient is taken to the theatre. The arm of the nightdress on the side where the operation is to be must not be put on—if the arm or breast is the affected part. Patients should always have on their stockings, and when flannel drawers can be worn, *without the slightest risk* of their proving inconvenient in the theatre, it may be done—for the twofold reason of avoiding all unnecessary exposure, and of keeping the patient warm. The patient's throat and neck should be kept quite free, and the nightdress unbuttoned or untied, as the case may be. It will mostly rest with the sister or nurse to place the mackintosh, and great care should be taken that this is done effectually, that the patient's clothing may not be unnecessarily soiled. The patients should always be carefully wrapped up whilst being conveyed to and from the theatre, to avoid their taking cold. Keep the parts that the surgeon is not immediately concerned with covered up in the theatre, that the vital powers may not be lowered unnecessarily by cold. You know that the tendency of anæsthetics is to reduce the temperature of the body. If the patient uses pins, or hair pins, habitually, you should persuade her to dispense with them on this occasion, as the patient frequently struggles violently in taking chloroform or ether, and they may hurt her or her attendants. You must also be careful to inquire if your patient has any false teeth, and see that they are removed prior to the operation.

But this is not quite all that a nurse should do for her patient by way of preparation, though perhaps it is all that can be technically demanded of her. I hope that none of *you* will feel that you have done your whole duty without sparing a little cheering and encouraging sympathy to help your patients through the ordeal awaiting them. It is a temptation, amidst the numberless cases which constantly fill the wards, for hospital nurses to forget that what is to them in hospital phraseology, " another breast case," " an amputation," and so on, is naturally a very different thing to the unfortunate patient who has to meet the trial in his own person. There is no harm in thinking and speaking of cases in this general sort of way, but it will be bad for yourselves in the end, as well as for the patients, if you lose your care and interest in the individual. Take care that you do not grow hardened in this way. There is no time to waste in much talking, neither is it necessary ; but the few minutes that you must bestow in preparing your patient in other ways will give the opportunity for the few encouraging words that means so much to them if they are spoken at the right time.

Try and put yourself in their place, and think as far as you can what you would like said to yourself on such an occasion. Never say what you do not believe to be true, but do take the trouble to say every encouraging thing that *is* true, and which can help the sufferer to look forward hope-

fully to the result. If you have known apparently similar
cases "get through" well, you can cheerfully mention the
fact. If you have reason to believe that the surgeon who is
to operate is specially clever, a quiet remark to that effect will
give the patient increased confidence. Never confide your
doubts and fears to a patient—that is not kind, nor necessary.
They may or may not be well founded, but you can do no
good by depressing the sufferer. Neither would it be right
to give false hopes; but you will earn much gratitude and be
doing right if you let your patients feel your interest in a
quiet womanly way, and surely it is a nurse's privilege " to
comfort and help the weak-hearted," as perhaps only she can
do on such occasions. Every one, almost without exception,
will be secretly craving for this sympathy, though perhaps
they may give no evidence of such being the case. For the
most part patients are very brave. Remember that I do not
want you to chatter a great deal, and talk too much to them
about their trouble, only just to do unto them as you would
yourself wish to be done by under similar circumstances.

The theatre should be kept fresh, though not cold. From
65° to 70° Fahr. is the range of temperature for ovariotomy
and lithotomy cases, but it is best to get directions from the
surgeon in each case, as it is one of the details about which
they frequently differ. The instruments do not, as a rule,
come within your province, but it is well for you to notice
them as you have opportunity. They should be covered with
a towel, that the patient may be spared the sight of them.

In those places where the needles are threaded by the
nurse, she must remember to have a good supply ready
threaded, with whatever sutures the surgeon has ordered. In
your dressing basket, or arranged on a table according to the
custom of the hospital, you must have a supply of lint, cotton
wool, strapping ready cut, bandages of all kinds, gutta
percha tissue, drainage tubes, pins, broad and narrow tape,

needles, and towels. You must also be provided with olive oil, carbolic oil, plenty of hot and cold water, which is usually supplied, ice, brandy, morphia, a feeder, spoon, and medicine glass. Also a ball and hypodermic syringe, in case either may be needed in an emergency. You will need plenty of empty receivers for the reception of pus, dead bone, etc. Never throw away any of these things until you have orders to do so. A towel, receiver, and sponge is needed for the vomiting which the anæsthetic nearly always produces. The patient's head must be turned on one side to allow the vomited matter to escape. A perfectly dry sponge may be asked for to place inside the ether inhaler, so a nurse had better have one at hand that has not been recently wetted.

Sponges must be thoroughly cleansed and wrung out of cold or iced water as dry as possible. This is best done in a towel. Some surgeons like their sponges wrung out in water of a higher temperature, but then special orders will be given. This is the chief part of the nurse's business, and it is most important to do it well. If the operation is done under the carbolic spray, the sponges, after being washed, must be wrung out in $\frac{1}{30}$ carbolic lotion, and the nurse must remember that, in addition to the mackintosh that covers the table, two mackintoshes in very good condition will be required to protect the patient from the moisture from the spray.

A nurse must always have ready a basin of water and a clean sponge, as it may be asked for at any moment, and is often finally required to wash away the traces of blood before the dressing is applied. Of course, in operations done anti-septically, instead of water this must be $\frac{1}{30}$ carbolic lotion, and for these cases the surgeons will require this to be ready from the beginning for them to dip their hands in.

Nurses are not there to *see* the operation, remember, but to make their presence realized by the perfectly quiet way in which all wants are foreseen or supplied. There must be no talking that can be dispensed with, even on business. Try to catch every hint or suggestion quickly; *never* get in the light. This is the time of all others for exercising quiet self-control and intelligent observation. These directions apply to *all* operations generally. For amputations, or where there is a probability of much bleeding, a tray with sawdust should be placed under the operation table ready for use. The nurse or probationer in the ward should always have the patient's bed prepared for his return, hot bottles and blankets at hand, all ready for use. Be prepared for the tendency to vomit, and also for any symptoms of collapse, or any cessation of breathing after the chloroform or ether. It is better for the patient to "come to" gradually, if possible; but if the return to consciousness is too long delayed, water and a towel must be flapped about the patient's face and neck.

After the patient has thoroughly recovered from the effects of the anæsthetic, a nurse should remember that he has been many hours without food, and see that he has suitable nourishment supplied as soon as it is allowed.

After all operations, hemorrhage must be carefully watched for. There is always a possibility of it. Only experience can teach you what is meant by "a little oozing," as it is called, and the beginning of more serious bleeding. Place a towel or a piece of lint under the wound, in addition to a mackintosh and draw-sheet; so that, if you are in doubt whether any stain is fresh or not, you can pull it on a little, leaving the wound to rest in a clean place, and then you can easily see if the bleeding is fresh.

If bleeding has begun, and the surgeon has to be called, do not hurry away with the soiled sheets, etc., so that if he desires to see the quantity of blood which the patient has lost, he may be able to do so. If you are asked as to the quantity, do not say "streams" of blood, etc., but try to give the supposed quantity as accurately as you can. Remember

that a little makes a great show on linen. Patients, even if
conscious in other respects, may be quite unaware that
bleeding is going on. If the patient can see for himself
when bleeding occurs, always impress upon him to let you
know instantly, without making him nervous or frightened
about it ; and, of course, do not *trust* to his doing so. Have
cold water, ice, warm water, sponges, and towels ready, in
addition to your usual dressing basket of lint, etc., and
have a fresh dressing ready to replace the one which will
probably have to be removed. Do not wait until the surgeon
appears before getting these things ready, as all delay is *most
serious*.

The method for arresting bleeding by compression of
the artery with the various kinds of tourniquets, with
perchloride of iron, and the actual cautery, will be described to you in detail later on—also the difference between
arterial and venous bleeding. If hemorrhage occurs from a
" stump," raise it, if possible, whilst waiting for the surgeons.
Have an empty receiver ready for clots of blood. Be exceedingly prompt, but do not get flurried, nor frighten the
patient. The less he or she sees of what is going on the
better ; and remember, he will keenly watch your manner, and
even the expression of your face, to try and ascertain if there
is any cause for alarm in a matter of such vital importance
to him.

Now we will go on with the subject of operations.

In amputation cases you will always have to watch carefully for bleeding ; so, in addition to the ordinary mackintosh
and draw-sheet, which you will, of course, leave under the
stump, it is well to have a towel or a thick fold of lint placed
so that you can easily draw it a little from time to time, and
ascertain if any fresh bleeding is going on. You must steady
the stump carefully with a piece of bandage over the pillows,
to prevent starting. You will need a cradle to keep off the

weight of the bedclothes, and these must be so placed that you can see the limb and watch for bleeding without disturbing the patient.

Sometimes an ice-bag is ordered to be applied over antiseptic or other dressings, to check the tendency to bleed, and in these cases you must be specially careful about changing it promptly, and never allow one to remain on for a single minute after the ice has melted.

You will observe as a curious fact that patients constantly complain of pain in those parts that have been amputated, and, unreasonable as it sounds, the pain that they complain of is very real. Remember to keep the patient warm and comfortable. Sometimes it is quite desirable to have a warm bottle put to one side, when an ice-bag is ordered for the other. A cradle is not conducive to the comfort of a patient, except so far as the injured limb is concerned, and a small blanket, under the cradle, should be wrapped over any other parts that are likely to suffer from cold.

In cases of excision of the breast you must remember that the arm of the side affected must be carefully bound down to the side, and that the patient must not be allowed to use it on any pretext whatever. The nurse must not forget that considerable hemorrhage may take place without being apparent under the large dressings frequently employed for these cases, so she must watch the more carefully on account of this difficulty, and should not fail to notice any change in the pulse, or any increasing pallor of the patient, which may indicate that bleeding is going on.

Cases of excision of tongue need very careful watching and constant attention. The nurse must endeavour to anticipate her patient's wants in every way, and not give him the exertion and excitement of trying to make himself understood. The patient must be kept quiet, and made warm and comfortable. He must be guarded from draughts, as there is a risk of pneumonia in these cases. The mouth must be gently, but effectually, swabbed out with some disinfecting fluid—usually Condy's fluid in some water—from time to time, but this should not be done with sufficient frequency to worry the patient. The mouth must also be rinsed out occasionally with the same fluid, and great pains taken to keep it as free from offensive discharge as possible. No nourishment must be given by the mouth until the doctor gives permission. Some surgeons allow a very small quantity of iced water to be given, but others do not approve of this. Again, some surgeons permit small pieces of ice to be folded in very soft muslin, and put in the patient's mouth; but this, also, you must never do without orders. At first the nourishment is usually prescribed in the form of nutrient enemata, and these must be given regularly.

The nursing of a case of cleft palate requires the greatest care in administering nourishment and in keeping the patient from speaking and crying, or the operation will speedily break down and prove useless. Some surgeons insist that milk, beef-tea, or any liquid diet they may order shall be carefully strained through muslin before it is given to the patient ; but it is not necessary to do this unless you receive special instructions on the point. The nurse must carefully watch that no bleeding is going on, as the patient may swallow the blood to a considerable extent, and there is the risk of choking. For the operation tiny pieces of sponge, fastened on little holders for the purpose, will be required, and it may be the duty of the nurse to provide the hare-lip pins. I have already told you that the strapping used for these cases has to be specially cut for the purpose. As the patient may not speak, a nurse should watch very carefully to anticipate his wants.

Both skill and great attention are required for the efficient nursing of tracheotomy cases, as the life of the patient in a

large measure depends upon the prompt assistance and unremitting care of the person in charge. With children it is
necessary to be doubly watchful, lest they pull out the tube
in a paroxysm of difficult breathing, or lie over it, and thus
prevent the access and escape of air to and from the lungs.
Grown-up patients are easier to nurse, because they are
generally able to understand their condition ; but in nursing
them also you must be careful to forestall their wants as
much as you possibly can, without waiting more than you
can help for them to tell you.

For a tracheotomy case you will require a tent for the
bed. This is frequently made of cotton sheeting, cut the
required shape, and it may be bound round with a little
scarlet braid to give the bed a brighter appearance. This
serves to keep away all draughts, and to preserve an equable
temperature in the immediate neighbourhood of the patient.
It also condenses the steam—for a steam-kettle is generally,
though by no means invariably, employed. A ward thermometer should be hung inside the tent, to insure the desired
temperature being maintained. Where no special orders are
given, this should be from 65° to 70° Fahr. The great object
in reference to the temperature which the nurse should keep
in view is maintaining it at all times, night and day, as
equal as possible. It is *variations* of temperature, either in
the direction of heat or cold, which have to be guarded
against. For this reason you should replenish the steam-
kettle with boiling water, so that the steam may be steadily
maintained without intermission, and not fill up the kettle
with cold or warm water, which must of necessity prevent a
supply of steam for an interval.

You must have at hand a basin of water, and sponges,
feathers, olive oil and glycerine, lint and cotton wool ; tape
or flat white elastic for fastening in the tube ; a receiver, in
case of sickness ; a soft towel and the tracheotomy instruments

should be close at hand, but out of the patient's reach, and covered up out of sight also. The neck must be kept thoroughly dry and clean in feeding the patient; milk is apt to spill, and becomes sour on the patient's skin, and possibly the moist atmosphere has a tendency to make the neck get sore. You will always be shown exactly what you are expected to do. Try and be most careful and intelligent in your observation and accurate in your report, for you can be of the greatest service; and, above all, if the outer tube comes out, or any other unfortunate accident happens, remember that *life* may *literally* depend upon your presence of mind, self-control, and promptitude. You will very soon learn how to remove, clean, and replace the inner tube with facility; but perhaps I should warn you always to replace this tube immediately, and never to let it be out longer than is needful for cleansing purposes. It may be that the patient may have the appearance of breathing better with the somewhat larger aperture, but this must not lead you to forget that if the outer tube becomes clogged with mucous, you have not the same power of removing and cleaning that, and the patient may thus very shortly be in danger of suffocation.

The only other detail it occurs to me to mention in connection with the tube, is the care you must exercise that it is not suddenly jerked or coughed out while you are renewing the tape or elastic with which it is fastened. You should, as far as may be practicable, pass the fresh tape or elastic through the fastening before removing the other. I have said that you will require feathers, and they must always be at hand, but their use should be restricted as far as possible. Some nurses get into a habit of poking feathers into the tube on all occasions, with more vigour than discretion, forgetting that such a proceeding is apt to irritate the trachea, and is, moreover, quite unnecessary. Nevertheless, a feather judiciously applied can be of great service in removing mucus that is clogging up the trachea and the entrance to the tube, and there *are* times when nothing else is equally well adapted for the purpose.

Sometimes small pieces of flannel wrung out of hot water are ordered to be placed across the tube. These fomentations must be frequently renewed, for of course they cannot be covered up with any waterproof material.

The three distinct objects which a nurse must always keep before her in taking charge of tracheotomy cases are— keeping the tube free from mucus; maintaining an equal temperature; and the careful support of the patients' strength by inducing them to take the nourishment ordered.

When you are nursing these cases, you must always be careful lest in attending to the patient you catch by accident any of the discharge, which is forced out from the tube with some violence, and which might be dangerous to you, should the case be of an infectious nature. I may also take this opportunity of reminding you that when you are nursing in this warm, moist atmosphere, you should be careful to wrap up before you leave the ward, and to keep out of draughts. You are likely to be more than usually susceptible to cold under such circumstances, and, knowing this, nurses should exercise some common sense for the preservation of their health. Be sure and get a walk every day before beginning your close attendance on these anxious but most interesting cases.

There are one or two duties that it is essential for a trained nurse to be able to perform efficiently, and I think perhaps it will be easier to explain them clearly as complete in themselves, than to break off in the midst of describing the nursing of any special case with a view of making the details to which I refer more clear to you.

I would first speak, then, of such offices as passing the

K

catheter, washing out the bladder, and syringing the vagina.
If you understand, to begin with, how these things should
be done, I shall only need briefly to refer to either process
afterwards, without lingering to explain it over again in
detail.

One practical illustration in the wards of how to introduce
the catheter will make it much more clear to you than any
theoretical description; but, as I do not like to pass the
subject over altogether, I will briefly quote the directions
which Dr. Smith gives on the matter.

"The patient should be placed upon her back, with the
knees drawn slightly up. The nurse should stand on the
right side, pass the left hand between the thighs, and place
the forefinger on the orifice of the vagina; the catheter can
then be readily introduced with the right hand, and being
made to glide over the finger of the left, will invariably enter
the urethra, and be felt through the walls of the vagina and
beneath the arch of the pubes, as it passes to the bladder."

I need scarcely remind you that this must always be done
with the utmost care and delicacy. You must *never* attempt
to pass the catheter merely for the sake of experience, nor
try to do so alone without the sister's permission, which of
course she will not give until she feels assured you are
competent to do it. Try in this, as in all your other work, to
make your patient the first consideration, and to render the
exposure necessary for your instruction as little distasteful to
them as possible. Only practice can enable you to perform
this without uncovering the patient, and you must never
attempt to do it in this way until you have become familiar
with this part of a nurse's duty.

After some operations it is by no means as easy to introduce the catheter as it is in the majority of cases, and unless
you observe carefully you may suppose the catheter has
reached the bladder when it has only passed into the vagina.

The catheter should not be introduced more than two inches, and no pressure or force should be employed under any circumstances. Experience will give you the necessary knowledge and confidence, as nothing else can, and the more you understand the more you will realize the necessity for taking pains to become efficient over all these details of trained nursing.

For passing the catheter the nurse should provide herself with a receiver for the urine, some olive oil—for of course the catheter must be well oiled before using—and a towel. Be sure and leave the patient perfectly dry and comfortable.

To wash out the bladder, and to inject some fluid into it, is sometimes an order which a nurse has to carry out. Extreme gentleness is necessary, for you may do serious injury by using the least force in any way. The neatest way is to have a full-sized catheter, or the end of a full-sized catheter with a piece of indiarubber tubing joined on, and a glass funnel fitted to the other end of the tube.

Of course you will first draw off any urine that may be in the bladder. Do not forget that the end of the catheter must be oiled before using, as much for this as for the ordinary purpose. It takes two to do this gently and efficiently, as it always should be done. One person to hold the funnel at the required height to pour in the fluid by degrees, and to let it escape slowly from the bladder from time to time by lowering the funnel into a vessel placed to receive the contents; the other to attend to the catheter, which must not be moved at all until the process is quite over. The other method of managing this is to put the end of the catheter on to a syringe. The objection to this is that the fluid is necessarily jerked in instead of flowing in steadily; but, as some doctors prefer it, it is well that you should be acquainted with both ways—remembering that when you have no distinct orders to the contrary, the former method is best.

In reference to vaginal injections, I cannot do better than quote the directions which Dr. Cullingworth gives in his "Manual of Nursing." He says, "They are usually administered by means of a Higginson's syringe, to which has been attached a vaginal tube. This tube, which should be made of hard rubber, is sold with the syringe; it is a straight tube five inches long, with a number of little holes pierced in the sides of its olive-shaped nozzle. . . . The proper mode of using it is as follows: The patient lies near the edge of the bed, on her back, with a round earthenware bed-pan underneath her to receive the returning fluid. The knees are drawn up; the nozzle of the tube, previously oiled or anointed with vaseline, is passed under the right knee and so into the vagina, the end being directed towards the upper and back part of the canal. The patient herself can hold this part of the apparatus in position, while the nurse, having placed the other end in the jug or basin which contains the fluid to be injected, and which has been conveniently arranged close to the side of the bed, gently compresses the pump of the syringe, allows it to refill, and empties it again, and so on until the desired quantity has been slowly injected. In withdrawing the nozzle, its point should be kept upwards to prevent what fluid remains in the apparatus from running out. The syringe, after being used, should be well cleansed and hung up by a loop tied round its metallic end. Almost any quantity can be injected by this method, the only limit being the size of the receptacle. A vaginal douche has this amongst other advantages, that a patient having once obtained the proper apparatus, can easily dispense with the services of an assistant. The best instrument for the purpose is one known as the irrigator. It consists of a tin pail or reservoir, capable of containing from one to four quarts of fluid, which is made to stand on a wall-bracket or chest of drawers, two or three feet above the level of the bed. At the side of the pail, near the bottom, is an opening into which is fixed the end of a long tube, furnished at its other extremity with a stop-cock, and terminating in a perforated nozzle of vulcanite, the perforations being at the sides of the nozzle and not at the tip.

"Vaginal injections may be simple or medicated. For cleansing purposes, either pure tepid (70° to 85° Fahr.) or warm (85° to 100° Fahr.) water may be used, or some disinfectant solution—*i.e.* Condy's fluid, in the proportion of a teaspoonful to each pint of warm water. Medicated injections are only to be given when ordered by the medical attendant, who will give all necessary directions for their use. Injections of pure hot water (100° to 110°, and even 115° Fahr.) have been recently much prescribed, especially for the relief of certain local inflammations."

The nursing of cases of ovariotomy, one of the most important operations of which you can ever have charge, will serve in a great measure as a type of all other abdominal sections, therefore we will enter fully into the nursing details connected with it. If we take this as the one for general guidance, it will be easy to distinguish afterwards the points of difference for the nursing of the varied abdominal operations. respectively.

Whether you are called to the nursing of a private case of ovariotomy, or whether you have the advantage of having the patient under intelligent supervision in a hospital, you will generally notice that she is recommended to live well and to keep as quiet and cheerful as possible for some days before the operation. Some doctors prefer the patient's temperature to be taken night and morning during this time. Unless it is known how the patient tolerates morphia, the surgeon occasionally orders one-sixth of a grain to be injected hypodermically prior to the operation, that he may see the effect. The patient should have a warm bath the night

before the operation, as it is very important she should get
no chill nor experience any unnecessary fatigue on the day.
Half an ounce of castor oil is usually given the night before,
and followed by a soap-and-water enema the next morning.
The enema is usually repeated about two hours before the
operation. The nurse should pass the catheter once or twice
beforehand to ensure the patient getting used to the process,
and this should be done about ten minutes before the operation. If this is to take place at two p.m. a good breakfast
should be given about six or half-past six a.m., and some
strong beef-tea, though nothing solid, should be given about
half-past nine a.m. The patient's hair should be well brushed
and plaited in two firm plaits, as it may be some time before
it can be properly brushed again, and arranging it in two
plaits not only makes it easier to brush without disturbing
the patient, but prevents her having a hard lump at the back
of the head to lie on. The patient should have on warm
woollen stockings, long enough to come well up over the
knees, a night-dress opening up the back for the convenience
of getting it out of the way, and a short flannel jacket fastening in the same way. When the patient is ready a light
blanket should be thrown over her until the operation begins.

You will take care that the patient does not see the preparations for the operation, nor is made conscious of them in any
way that can be avoided. You must have ready a mackintosh
and blanket for the operating-table, a smaller mackintosh
with an oval aperture the size of the proposed incision, with
a circle of strapping gummed, or better still, sewn on to the
under side of the mackintosh, with the adhesive side left free
to attach it to the patient. All the water and carbolic lotion
used will be required warm. Everything used in connection
with this operation should, if possible, be perfectly new. Allow
no sponge to be in the room except the new ones that have
been carefully prepared for the case, and *accurately counted.*

If the surgeon is in any doubt as to whether all the sponges have been removed from the wound it will be a satisfaction to him to have this fact ascertained beyond all possibility of doubt by having the sponges counted. About twenty sponges are sufficient. There should be two rather large flat sponges for pressing the abdomen, six or eight small ones on sponge-holders, and the remainder should be of the size usually employed in the theatre. You should keep one clean sponge apart from the others, with some $\frac{1}{30}$ carbolic lotion in readiness to wash round the wound in the end. I should mention that $\frac{1}{30}$ carbolic lotion is used for everything, including the washing of sponges, except for the spray, for dipping the instruments in before using, and for washing the surface where the incision is to be made prior to the operation. This should be done by the nurse immediately prior to the operation, but in most cases the surgeon will ask for it to be done again in his presence, and he will require some carbolic lotion ready for him to dip his hands into before he commences. You should have a little chloroform ready on some lint to wipe off the marks of the strapping before the usual antiseptic dressing is applied. You should have in readiness plenty of dry gauze pads of all sizes, a roll of boracic lint, a wide flannel binder, say a yard and a half long by half a yard wide, with a square of double lint sewn over the portion that covers the back to prevent the flannel chafing the skin. Some surgeons prefer a linen binder sewn outside the flannel to give a firmer support, but you would not do this without orders, which, indeed, should always be given or asked for in every instance. Occasionally a T bandage is employed to keep the dressing in place. You will require *new* fomentation flannels and wringers, three empty buckets to receive the fluid, or perhaps more; at least two carbolic basins and a white receiver. You should also have at hand, brandy, morphia, and the syringes required for injecting them, morphia suppositories, ammonia, ice, and safety pins; in short, the usual things required for operations, with the addition of those that I have specially mentioned. You will have warm towels in readiness in case they are asked for. The temperature of the room is usually about 68° or 70° Fahr. when you receive no distinct orders.

The bed for a case of ovariotomy requires to be specially made. There should, if possible, be two hair mattresses, or, at any rate, you must ensure a sufficient thickness to protect the patient from any discomfort arising from coming in too close contact with the bedstead. Over the bottom sheet you should put a mackintosh and draw-sheet. There should be two soft pillows for the patient's head and shoulders, and one firm pillow to support the knees, and thus relieve all strain from the abdominal muscles. There should be a square water pillow, just warm, and not filled too full, placed ready for the patient's back, and hot water bottles should also be ready for use. As a rule, nothing cold is allowed to come near the patient except the ice that she is usually ordered to suck. In some hospitals a cradle is used as a matter of routine for ovarian cases, and in others it is only employed if the patient is suffering from peritonitis, or finds the weight of the bed-clothes an inconvenience. Either way the upper bedclothes are made to open in the middle. To do this neatly you require two top sheets, and two top blankets. These should be doubled and placed so that they meet in the middle of the bed. In this way all unnecessary exposure of the patient is avoided. The check must be put on over this in the usual way, and of course it has to be doubled back when the clothes have to be moved aside.

I am not sure if this description conveys a clear idea to your mind, but I cannot explain it better without giving you a practical illustration on a bed, and this you will doubtless soon get in the wards. The catheter must be passed every six hours, oftener if necessary. A specimen of the urine must be saved, and the quantity measured. The temperature is usually taken every four hours unless the patient is sleeping, and the nurse is sometimes expected to take the pulse and respiration night and morning. The nurse may give *nothing* by the mouth—sometimes even ice is forbidden —until she has permission to do so. The surgeon will give orders on this point, and also tell you when to begin the nutrient enemata. These must be injected very gently and lukewarm. The patient is frequently troubled with flatulency, and if you are giving the nutrient enema with a catheter and a ball syringe in the way I have previously described to you, it is best to pass the catheter into the rectum before attaching it to the tube of the syringe, so that any wind may be allowed to escape. Attention to this detail may not only relieve the patient, but may make the difference of the nourishment given being retained or returned.

The bed must, of course, be kept scrupulously clean, smooth, and fresh; but there must be as little moving or changing of the patient as is consistent with attaining this object. Ovarian cases must not be turned on their sides in the usual way for changing the sheets of helpless patients, but the draw-sheet—the only part of the bedding that it should be necessary to change at first—should be securely pinned to the one that is about to be removed, and in this way it can easily be drawn through if the nurse gently inserts her hands under the patient's back and raises her —not more than two inches—while the assistant attends to the sheet. I need scarcely pause to remind you that one person must never attempt to change the under sheet of an ovarian case without help. The fresh bedding as well as all changes of body linen should be put on warm, and chills carefully guarded against. In all probability the bowels will not act for some days, and then it will be safe for the patient to be raised on to the bed-pan. This must be warmed with hot water prior to use, to avoid all shock from the patient coming in contact with the cold earthenware, and a little oil should be rubbed round the edges to facilitate its readily slipping into position if the patient perspires.

If there is any tendency to bed-sores a piece of oiled lint or simple dressing can be gently inserted under the flannel binder to keep the patient's back from getting rubbed. Much of the success of the case, and a great deal of the comfort of the patient, depends upon the perfect stillness in one position, *i.e.* lying on the back with the knees drawn up for the first few days. If the patient vomits, sneezes, or coughs, the nurse must place her hand gently over the region of the incision to give firm support, and keep up a steady pressure until the patient is quiet again. You must spare no pains to induce her to lie as still as possible. The most careful observation and accurate reports are expected from the nurse. You cannot be too exact about every detail. The atmosphere surrounding the patient must be kept as fresh and as free from every bad smell as you can manage to have it, for the welfare of these critical cases greatly depend upon their surroundings. There must always be a ward thermometer in the room, and the nurse must be careful to maintain the temperature ordered. You will probably find that this varies to a considerable extent; some surgeons preferring a high temperature and plenty of hot bottles, and others being of opinion that too much heat exhausts the patient's strength, but on such points you can always ask for instructions, and then obediently carry them out.

I believe that is all which it occurs to me to tell you in reference to these cases. I will refer to the others more briefly.

Hernia cases require the bed made in the way just described. The patient must be kept lying on her back, and for this reason you will need to pass the catheter. The

affected part must be carefully supported by the hand during
all convulsive movements in the manner I have just spoken
of. No solid food must be given, but as the feeding is
important you must be careful to induce the patient to take
the nourishment ordered, night and day. Ice is nearly
always prescribed for these cases. The doctor may wish to
see the vomited matter, as well as the motions.

Lithotomy cases also need the bed made with the divided
upper bedclothes in the manner that you now understand.
The nurse's chief anxiety in these cases is the prevention of
bedsores, and the difficult task of keeping the bed as dry,
clean, and as free from smell as possible. It is also important
to remember that nothing cold comes near him, that sheets
and blankets, however frequently they may be changed, must
always be warm. Some surgeons will only permit pieces of
old blankets to be used as draw-sheets, but others have no
objection to ordinary draw-sheets, provided they are always
kept dry and warm.

Sponges are required to absorb the urine, which will at first
flow through the wound. These must be kept scrupulously
clean, and frequently changed. They should be wrung out
in *cold* water and carbolic acid, not warm water, as it increases
the smell. They should be squeezed perfectly dry, to render
them capable of absorbing as much urine as possible, and so
that you may be able to judge pretty accurately how much
urine passes through the wound. The surgeon will expect
the nurse to be able to tell him when the urine begins to flow
through the natural orifice, and also when it ceases to flow
through the wound. Any appearance of blood in the urine
must be at once reported to the surgeon.

There are various methods of arranging the under part
of the bed for lithotomy cases. Proper mattresses, with a
hole in the centre, in which a vessel can be placed to receive
the urine, are made expressly for this purpose. This should

be covered with a mackintosh, made also with a hole in the
centre, and placed in a manner to conduce to the comfort of
the patient, and to protect the mattress.

The nurse must be especially careful that the patient does
not take cold from the washings near the wound, which will
be needed to keep the skin from getting sore. Every conceivable precaution must be taken against bed-sores. The
surrounding parts should be smeared with some greasy substance to resist the moisture, such as vaseline, gall ointment,
zinc dressing, or anything that may be considered equally
suitable for the purpose. I am sure you will all recognize
the necessity of making a patient in this distressing condition
as comfortable as you can. You must keep a careful look
out for hemorrhage or rigors. The occurrence of either
must be promptly reported to the surgeon. I should mention
that, in cases of lithotomy, lithotrity, and stricture, the blanket
which the nurse has in reserve to cover the patient after the
operation should be warm.

The only point to which I need call your attention in
cases of lithotrity is that the surgeon will expect all the urine
to be carefully measured and strained, and all the fragments
of stone reserved for his inspection. When you have charge
of stricture cases you must guard against chills, see that the
bed and body linen of your patient is supplied warm, and
watch carefully for rigors.

In most uterine operations the special point you have to
keep in remembrance is that the patient must not be allowed
to stand or sit up for some days, though in other respects she
may feel and be quite well.

There are one or two details that perhaps I should mention
in connection with cases of ruptured perinæum. Most
surgeons prefer the knees to be tied together, but that is
a matter for them to decide, and you will merely be careful
that their wishes are carried out. The patient lies on her

side, and may be gently turned from one side to the other to suit her inclination. The catheter must be passed regularly, and care taken to avoid any drops of urine getting into the wound. The bowels are kept persistently confined. If there is any inclination for the bowels to act before the doctor considers it desirable, morphia suppositories are usually ordered. These should be thoroughly and effectually passed up the rectum. This is best done by gently pushing them in with a well-oiled catheter or bougie, and thus you avoid distending the anus with the finger, as is sometimes done. The patient is not allowed solid food. When the doctor wishes the bowels to be opened, enemas as well as aperients are usually prescribed. An oil enema first generally helps to produce a satisfactory result if you are permitted to give it. You must on no account leave your patient a moment alone at this critical time. It may be necessary to support the perinæum, and the patient often suffers much pain.

It is possible that as private nurses you may be sent to take charge of ophthalmic operations, and as many of you may not have met with any in your experience in the general wards, I will just mention one or two particulars for your guidance.

Cataract is the most important eye operation with regard to nursing, as its success greatly depends on the care of the nurse. It is very important that the patient's general health should be in as good a condition as possible; therefore, if you have charge of the patient for some time before the operation, see that he is as well nourished, and that he gets as much fresh air as possible.

You must take especial care to cheer your patients, and remember that their condition of blind helplessness is very depressing. The more they have learnt to like and trust the nurse, the more service she will be able to render them; and when you reflect that the sight may be lost for ever through carelessness on your part, I am sure you will spare no effort to ensure a good result.

Before the operation, see that the patient's head, face, and neck are absolutely clean, the hair brushed back from the face and, if long, plaited in two plaits, as the patient will not be able to be washed or the hair brushed for a week. In other ways the patient is prepared for the operation in the usual manner.

Small, fine sponges will be needed at the operation. After the operation the eyelid will be strapped down with two small pieces of strapping. It is best to smear the eyebrows with olive oil before doing this. Both eyes should be covered with lint and cotton-wool, and bandaged firmly, then place the patient in bed entirely in the dark.

Do all you can to obviate the tendency to sickness for the first twenty-four hours. The patient must lie on his back for the first four days. Unless otherwise ordered, give a nourishing slop diet for the first eight days. When other food is allowed, be careful that no hard crusts, etc., are given, or anything that it would cause the patient the least effort to bite.

In cases of cataract no opiates or alcohol must be given without express orders. If the patient complains of much pain soon after the operation, and if there is much swelling of the eyelid, you will usually be told to apply a leech over the temple, otherwise it is best not to touch the bandage until the next day. Then repeat the same dressing that was applied at the operation, very gently wiping the eyelid with damp cotton-wool, and drawing down the lower lid to let any tears escape. You must notice the quantity of discharge to report to the surgeon. As a rule, if the eyes are doing well, there will be little or no discharge, and not much pain after the first twenty-four hours. On the eighth day the eye which has not been operated upon may be uncovered, but the other eye must be treated as before until the surgeon has seen it. You will please observe carefully that these suggestions are merely for your guidance when no orders are given, but be exceedingly exact about obtaining and carrying out any instructions you can get from the individual surgeon whose case you may be nursing.

In cases of iridectomy (double) both eyes must be covered up for a week. Then, as a rule, they may be uncovered, and only a shade worn. They may be bathed with tepid or cold water twice a day from the day after the operation.

In cases of iridectomy (single) both eyes must be tied up at first with double lint and cotton-wool, but the one may be uncovered the following day if the patient keeps in a dull light for a week.

I think, after what I have said, you will soon learn all that is needful for you to know in connection with the innumerable minor operations, that are constantly coming before you in the wards.

LECTURE VIII.

IN the beginning of these lectures we considered the distinction between the nurse's work and the doctor's, and the relation which they bear to each other in their work. I think we have clearly kept before us the leading idea that it is the doctor's part to lay down a system of scientific treatment, and yours to be the active agents in carrying this plan of treatment into effect. You have also been told that treatment usually presents itself under one or more of three aspects.

First, it may be necessary to provide an antidote to any poison, and to remove all sources of harm; secondly, the chief consideration may be to place and to keep the patient in the most favourable condition for self-cure; thirdly, it may be desirable to aid in treatment by drugs which experience or experiment have shown to be efficacious. It is under this, the third heading, that the subject of to-night's lecture comes.

Already we have discussed somewhat minutely the nurse's duties in connection with the forms of treatment spoken of under headings one and two. We have considered all that is important for a nurse in keeping her patient perfectly at "rest," i.e. of applying the treatment of "rest," general and partial. We have also spoken in detail of the application, both general and partial, of such natural agents as heat and cold. Now we come to the complicated subject of "drugs," for it certainly is more difficult for a nurse to acquire, or even to know what *is* the sort and extent of the knowledge necessary or useful for her to acquire in this branch of treatment.

Drugs—by that we understand the ingredients used for making up medicine—are prescribed for the cure or relief of disease. When we say the cure of disease, we mean really the putting of the body into such a condition as will enable it to recover itself—we do *not* mean that the drug directly cures the ailment in question.

By medicine we mean *any* remedy given internally, in whatever form; therefore it is not accurate for a nurse to say, "this patient has not had his medicine, but I have just given him a pill, or a powder." Nurses sometimes get into a way of thinking that the term medicine only applies to a draught or a mixture.

Drugs may be employed for one of three objects—

1st. As a direct antidote for some poison, as, for example, chalk is given for oxalic acid poisoning.

2nd. To produce effects which *experiment* has proved they will do—as, for example, digitalis (which is a preparation of the ordinary foxglove, as some of you know) is definitely known to produce distinct effects for certain affections of the heart.

3rd. To produce effects which *experience* has shown they will do, apart from experiment; and we may take the familiar example of a cup of tea as a remedy for some sorts of headache. We know it *will* in many cases have the desired effect, but of this and many other remedies, doctors can only tell us that experience proves it, they cannot explain *why*, nor demonstrate the fact definitely by experiment. This last is called empiricism, or empirical treatment. I need scarcely say that I do not wish any of you to take to talking about empiricism or empirical treatment, but they are terms that you will so frequently hear used, that you may as well understand what is meant by them.

L

As scientific knowledge increases, the first and second objects for which drugs are employed are developed. New antidotes for poisons are discovered, and experiments almost daily increase the knowledge of what effects can be produced in that direction.

It is under the third heading—drugs given to produce effects that experience and not experiment has proved they will do—which has constituted the bulk of drug treatment hitherto, though the vast numbers of drugs that were formerly employed are now much reduced, and many in general use at an earlier period are now never heard of.

Much of the effect of drugs will depend on the circumstances under which they are given. Whether before or after meals. The state of the patient's health also influences the effects of drugs. In addition to this there are special idiosyncrasies of individuals—some cannot tolerate opium, for example—to be taken into consideration.

Doctors acknowledge this to be a branch which requires much more information, and from the doubt about the effect of remedies springs many differences of opinion. The very nature of the question renders it difficult if not impossible to arrive at definite conclusions that can be accepted equally by all. The public have great, almost unlimited, faith in drugs, as is illustrated by quack remedies, and the abounding popularity of them.

As a rule, drugs are given with a view of getting them into the blood and circulating to the different organs. Sometimes they are given for their local action only. Drugs have specific action, i.e. some act as antidotes for some poisons, some act as tonics, aperients, expectorants, sedatives, and narcotics, some cause sweating, some act as stimulants, some as astringents, and arrest hemorrhage, some as emetics.

Medicines are prepared in a variety of forms, and may be administered in the shape of draughts, small doses, pills, powders, or lozenges. Formerly the most nauseous compounds were prescribed and swallowed as a matter of course, but latterly much pains has been taken to make drugs available in the most effective and palatable form which can be devised. If you compare the well-known brimstone and treacle, for instance, to the perfectly prepared pills and lozenges of to-day, you cannot fail to see what an advance has taken place in this respect.

Now, drugs are introduced into the system by the mouth in the various forms referred to; by the rectum, as in the form of enemas, or suppositories; by hypodermic injections, by inhalation, and also by absorption through the skin.

The nurse's work in connection with drugs lies chiefly in their accurate and skilful administration; and there is also much room for a nurse to aid by most careful observation of the effects produced, as she has the best opportunity for noting them.

It can scarcely be necessary for me to impress upon you the paramount importance of absolute *accuracy* in the measurement of any medicine you give, whatever form it may have to be administered in. You are well aware that in some instances a slight inaccuracy may cause fatal results; in other cases it may not be of much consequence; but the *habit* of perfect accuracy is all important—absolutely essential—to good nursing.

You should all learn the simple table of English measurements, if you do not already know it. I mean the following:—

One minim = one drop.
Sixty minims = one fluid drachm (one teaspoonful).
Eight fluid drachms = one fluid ounce (two tablespoonfuls).
½ ounce = one tablespoon or four teaspoonfuls.
Twenty fluid ounces = one pint.

And be sure you thoroughly understand the measure glasses; notice them again and again, until you are as confident that you understand them as you are that you know the difference between an ordinary tea and table spoon. Carelessness in this respect is unpardonable, and the possible consequences of error are terrible to think of. It is hopeless for a doctor to form a correct estimate of the effects, if his prescriptions are not rightly given according to orders. *Always* read the label, no matter how familiar you may imagine that you are with it. Almost every hospital has its sad story of accidents —which might so easily have been prevented—from neglect of this simple rule.

This is another habit you must resolve to, cultivate for yourselves : carefully shake up those mixtures that have thick sediments at the bottom of the bottle, and do not pour the dose into the glass until you are close to the patient, and he is quite ready to swallow it. Do not leave bottles uncorked. Impress upon your patients that if they do not wish to taste their medicine much, they must avoid touching it *with their lips,* and take care they have a handkerchief or something at hand to wipe their lips at once. This precaution will often prevent the medicine being vomited by patients who are inclined to sickness. Never make your patient drink off an unpalatable draught when his lips, mouth, and throat are dry and ready to absorb quickly the first liquid that comes in contact with them. He will taste it much less if his mouth is moistened previously.

In considering all these details, your chief object is to get the medicine taken properly, with as little discomfort to the patient as care and skill can secure. There is much scope for the " art " of nursing to be cultivated in this direction, and you will not only spare your patients much that is disagreeable, but may ensure greater success in efficiently carrying out treatment, if you excel in the administration of medicine.

Between the doctor thinking of and prescribing a certain

drug, and the nurse getting that drug into the patient, there is a considerable interval, and often the difficulties of carrying out these orders are not much taken into consideration by the doctor. You must study in each instance the best way of meeting and conquering these difficulties. Not only children, but adults—those who are conscious, as well as delirious patients—will often refuse remedies from one and take it readily from another. Why?

It is not only a difference in manner, but it is partly owing to care in such details as the perfect cleanliness of the glass—the avoidance as much as possible of forcing the disagreeable smell upon your patient—by poking the glass straight under his nose while you are persuading him to take it, more especially if the odour is as offensive as that of valerian, asafœtida, etc. The usual method of giving medicines round the ward with a basin of water and towel is very good; but in this case leave any disagreeable smelling medicines to be given last, and do not victimize *all* the patients unnecessarily with the discomfort of having an offensive odour added to that of their own medicine. Do not give effervescing medicines in too small a glass, and make the patient or bed in a mess, nor pour it out in such a way as to let all the effervescence go off before the patient can sit up. Of course, if the patient will not drink it in a state of effervescence, you cannot help it, but take care that he has the chance.

Oils are the medicines most objected to, as a rule, and they should be given with great nicety. They are best floated on the top of some liquid—brandy, coffee, beef-tea, milk. Follow the inclination of the patient in these details. Wash the glass well round with the chosen liquid, and then pour the oil carefully in the centre of it. Castor oil is best given on an empty stomach; and this is the general rule for most purgatives. It is said that hot beef-tea, made very salt, disguises the taste of castor oil better than anything else; and

this is the liquid I would recommend to you for the purpose.   But in this instance the oil should be completely and
thoroughly beaten up with the beef-tea, and not floated on
the top of it.   Cod liver oil is best given *immediately* after
food.   It is usually taken without any of the vehicles employed for castor oil.   Croton oil is comparatively rarely used.
The dose is from half a minim to six minims : it is given in
butter or on sugar.

Iron and arsenic are always best given after meals.   I
mention this, though directions for hours and quantity are
nearly always given in each case.   Ten, two, and six are the
most convenient times for four hour and " three times a day "
medicines when no orders are given.

Pills should be given in any way to suit the patient.
Large pills are easier to swallow than small ones.   Powders
must also be mixed to suit the cases ; for small children
moisten your finger so that the powder can adhere to it, and
place it well back on the tongue.   After administering emetics
you must have a vessel ready for sudden speedy results.

Now, in order to report fully and carefully the effects of
medicines, a nurse must understand to some extent the object
for which they are given, if only the broad classification of
aperients, tonics, astringents, narcotics, sedatives, and so on.

It is almost dangerous to tread upon ground so nearly
bordering on the line of where doctor's work begins and
nurses' work ends.   Nevertheless, I recommend you to study
some of the known effects of certain drugs, with a strong
warning that any such knowledge is for guidance, and not
for display, nor even for remark.   Do not say to the doctor,
for instance, " I thought I had better tell you such and such
a symptom, etc., because the patient is taking such and
such a drug."   With a few definite things you may imply
that, as aperients and narcotics, for instance, are given for
a distinct and visible object; but you must carefully avoid

this where the effects intended to be reached are more obscure. It looks officious and ignorant not only in knowledge of drugs, but ignorant of the nurse's place and training, which is far more deplorable.

When you have become acquainted with the effects of any drugs, note for yourselves what you see of them in practical use, and report their *effects* simply, without comment in any shape as to what cause these effects may be due. The chief object in view is to prevent the doctor remaining in ignorance of them. If you perceive certain things, and believe them due to certain causes, of course you will not alter the treatment on your own responsibility, but you will take care that the doctor is duly informed before you continue it, and then you will have thoroughly done your part as an intelligent help.

The giving of hypodermic injections is not likely to fall to your share, until you have become much more experienced; but it is well to make yourselves as familiar as possible with the process, and for this reason you should notice how it is done when opportunities occur. Practical illustrations are worth a great deal of theoretical instruction on this point.

Hypodermic is a Greek term, meaning " under the skin." The Latin term " subcutaneous " means the same thing. To give a hypodermic injection, pinch up a fold of the skin, firmly thrust the point of the syringe in, horizontally, after having dipped it in oil, and then slowly inject the fluid. In filling the syringe be *exceedingly* careful that no air gets mixed with the fluid. The orifice is so minute that the liquid will not generally escape, but it is as well to keep your finger on the spot for a minute when you withdraw the syringe. The quantity injected is always so small that the solutions used for the purpose are very powerful.

I need scarcely point out, and yet I must not fail to remind you, how quickly fatal any mistake as to the quantity

or strength of the liquid employed would almost inevitably
be. The greatest care and most minute accuracy are indispensable. In many hospitals the doctors will not permit
hypodermic injections to be administered by any but themselves, but other doctors think that there is no reason why
very experienced nurses should not be allowed to give them,
if they have been shown how, and are thoroughly trustworthy.

The custom in this hospital, as most of you are aware, is
for the sisters to give hypodermic injections whenever they
are ordered. No nurse or probationer is allowed to do so,
and I am glad to take the opportunity of making all new-
comers distinctly acquainted with this rule. At the same
time I am always glad when the night or day sisters give
you instructions on the point, and when they permit any one,
who appears to them sufficiently capable, to give the hypodermic injection in their presence. But you must not allow
the fact of your knowing how to do this, individually, interfere
with the general rule that no nurse or probationer here is
permitted to give the hypodermic injections, and you will
remember that you have no right under any circumstances to
take upon yourselves the responsibility of making an exception to an established custom in this hospital. This fact is
no argument to prevent each one of you acquainting yourselves with this method of administering drugs, every time
that you have the opportunity. Be sure, too, that you learn
to read the hypodermic syringe correctly, that there may be
no possibility of error when it does fall to your share to give
a hypodermic injection elsewhere.

One grain of morphia in six minims is a common strength,
and two minims, that is, the third of a grain, is very generally prescribed, but implicit obedience to directions is all
important in every case.

In giving a hypodermic injection care must be taken to
avoid putting the syringe into a vein.

The fine point of a hypodermic syringe easily gets clogged up, especially when the gelatine discs have been employed for the injection, and it is then of no further use. To avoid this you must be particular to clean it *at once*, before the fluid into which it has been dipped has had time to dry on. Take care to pass some clean cold water once or twice through it, and it is a good plan when possible to keep a small piece of silver wire through the point when it is not in use. With careful usage a hypodermic syringe will keep in working order for some time, but not otherwise.

Brandy and other stimulants are sometimes injected hypodermically, but this is almost always done by the doctor. A larger syringe is, of course, required for this purpose.

Putting drops into the eye is a little matter that you may often have to attend to. I mention it in order to call your attention to the fact that anything dropped into the eye should be put in at the outside corner, not the side next to the nose. The reason for this is that in the outside corner of the eye there is a gland continually secreting and pouring out a fluid we call *tears*. This fluid lubricates the surface of the eyeball, and then runs down a little tube, whose orifice we can see at the inner corner of our eyes, into the nose. Consequently, anything dropped into the outside corner of the eye will suffuse itself over the surface on its way to the little tube before mentioned, and that is what you want the drops to do.

Mortar or lime in the eye occasions great pain, and injury also, if it is not speedily removed. If you have it to deal with *immediately*, the eye should be well washed with a tepid solution of vinegar and water (about a teaspoonful of vinegar to two ounces of water). The lid should be everted, and all particles must be gently removed. A drop or two of castor oil dropped into the eye after it has been irritated will greatly soothe it.

Many drugs now employed for inhalation are administered

on a piece of lint placed in a wire respirator, and worn by the patient constantly or according to orders.

Another method liked by some physicians is to heat a small pot by burning the methylated spirit inside it, and directly this has burnt out, pouring the exact quantity of the prescribed drug on the hot surface and allowing the patient to inhale the fumes thus immediately thrown off.

In speaking of inhalations I must not omit to mention a very important drug, nitrate of amyl, which is occasionally employed in angina pectoris and other serious cases. It is an extremely powerful remedy, and must only be administered in strictest obedience to orders.

The correct doses of nitrate of amyl are prepared in little glass capsules to ensure the exact quantity being given, and as an effectual way of excluding this preparation from the air. When required for use the capsule is wrapped up in a piece of lint, promptly crushed by your foot or in any other convenient way, and then given to the patient to inhale from the lint.

Inhalations are given in various contrivances made for the purpose. Some are fatiguing, inasmuch as they necessitate the patient keeping his mouth over the tube or mouth of the vessel, and taking a distinct breath for the purpose of inhaling the vapour. A better invention, used in some hospitals, is Siegel's spray, for the purpose of impregnating the atmosphere immediately surrounding the patient's mouth, which enables him to inhale it without effort. Various drugs are used for inhalations. Take care not to scald the patient, either through the carelessness of having the steam too near at a scalding temperature, or from having the whole apparatus upset by him in a sudden struggle for breath or a violent cough. Watch for faintness in some cases. Inhalations of poppy-head water induce drowsiness. Patients should carefully avoid breathing cold air afterwards.

The most critical inhalations are those used as anæsthetics, such as ether, chloroform, and others, but of these we will speak in connection with their use at operations.

The absorption of drugs by the skin is a fact that it is important you should be aware of, when you have orders to use external applications containing mercury, opium, and any other drugs equally likely to produce a serious effect upon the system, so that you may be careful as to the quantity applied at any one time.

We have yet to speak of the introduction of drugs into the system through the rectum.

Suppositories are small conical preparations of various compounds, which are inserted into the rectum or the vagina. They act as astringents, and check the action of the bowels, or they relieve pain. Patients can often apply these themselves; but if there is any difficulty, the nurse must do it for them. You have only to dip your finger and the suppository into some oil, and introduce the suppository as far up as you conveniently can.

Enemas are of various kinds, and given for various purposes. They are used to procure the evacuation of the bowels, for the relief of pain, for restraining diarrhœa and dysentry, and for introducing medicine, stimulants, and nourishment into the system, when it is impossible, or deemed undesirable, to administer them in any other way. When an enema is given to relieve the bowels, a copious injection must be used. It usually consists of about a pint or more of warm water, with sufficent soap rubbed down in it to render it creamy. Soft soap is useful for the purpose, and prepares quickly. The usual proportion is about two ounces of soft soap to a pint of water. If a stronger remedy is required, half an ounce or an ounce of castor oil or turpentine is generally ordered, and this, mixed with a small quantity of gruel, or of the soap and water, should be placed in a separate vessel, and injected *first*, the remainder of the enema should immediately follow it, without the nozzle of the tube being removed from the rectum.

In this way the most important part of the remedy will be effectually given, whereas, if you attempt to mix the castor oil or the turpentine with the full quantity of soap and water, you will find that the castor oil or the turpentine, being lighter than the water, will float on the top, however well mixed it may be to begin with, and the chances are that the quantity ordered will never be given at all. Moreover, you will not easily cleanse the vessel, nor get rid of the smell of the castor oil, if you attempt to make one large mixture of it. Sometimes olive oil is ordered, and that should be given in the same way, as oil and water do not amalgamate. For giving these enemas, I have no hesitation in saying that a Higginson's syringe is quite the best apparatus. Various tubes are recommended for the purpose, and used at different hospitals.

Under all circumstances, and whatever appliance you may be using, take care that the part to be introduced into the rectum is thoroughly well oiled. It is inexcusable for a nurse to forget or lazily to neglect this, and I have heard with regret that there *are* nurses who are either so careless that they do not take the trouble or are so ignorant that they have not learnt the necessity of it. Please remember that this is a rule without an exception. On no account whatever must any force be used in introducing the mouth-piece into the rectum, even if any obstruction exists. The enema tube should not be introduced more than two or two and a half inches. In giving an enema a nurse should have at hand, in addition to the materials used for the enema, some utensil and cover in readiness, and a towel. The patient should, whenever possible, lie on the left side, near the edge of the bed, with the knees drawn up.

In removing the syringe, take care not to soil the sheet with some of the contents, and promptly roll the towel up, and press it against the patient to assist in retaining the enema for a few minutes, and this little attention is particularly necessary with children. Of course, if the fluid is permitted to return at once, it is likely to do so without producing a satisfactory result.

Dr. Smith states, in his very useful "Lectures on Nursing," that the temperature of the injection should be about 85° Fahr. Miss Wood says, in her "Handbook of Nursing," from 96° to 100° Fahr. The latter is a higher temperature than is usually given, and at any rate be very careful *never* to exceed that. I have heard of disastrous results ensuing from a nurse administering an enema hotter than it could safely be given.

Enemas to check diarrhœa are made of starch, usually with the addition of ten or twenty drops of laudanum, according to orders. Dr. Smith considers that starch enemas should be given at a temperature of 100° Fahr.; but that is a higher temperature than is recommended by most, and you will find in the majority of cases it is usual to administer starch enemas very cool indeed. I dare say most of you know that nearly all remedies for diarrhœa are given cold. The quantity should not exceed from one to two and a half ounces, unless special orders are given. As you will probably make rather more than the quantity you mean to give, take care to measure out the exact amount before adding the laudanum, otherwise a portion of it will be wasted, and the patient will not have the benefit of the full dose ordered.

Once more I must repeat my warning in reference to the effect of opium on children, and impress upon you the necessity for extreme caution when it is ordered for them. For children starch enemas are frequently ordered without any laudanum, or in very small quantities; but I am anxious

that you should realize the importance of the strictest adherence to orders, in this matter especially, both with regard
to time and quantity.

Starch enemas must be administered very slowly and
gently, with a view to causing as little disturbance as
possible. External pressure with the towel in the way I
have just described will sometimes be of great assistance
to the patient in retaining them, especially with children.
In many books you will find instructions to prepare starch
enemas with cold water, and, of course, when any doctors for
whom you are nursing prefer having them made in that way,
you will obediently carry out their orders. Otherwise you
will find that starch enemas made with boiling water are
more effectual, and this is the method given in the British
Pharmacopœia. The preparation must then be allowed to cool
down to the required temperature, and in some cases that
will be quite cold.

The best appliance for giving starch enemas is a glass
syringe. It is infinitely superior to the ball syringe, for
several reasons. You can *see* that no air is being given, either
before or after the mixture you are injecting; you can judge
more accurately how much has been given, if the patient
cannot receive it all, and there is no risk of the fluid being
drawn back into the tube again, as is sometimes the case with
the ball syringe. You also avoid the waste consequent upon
putting a small quantity of a somewhat sticky compound into
an unnecessarily large space.

It is also a very neat and clean arrangement. The part
introduced into the rectum must, of course, be oiled, and care
taken to hold the glass syringe firmly in the left hand, that
in slowly pressing the piston down with the right hand all
pressure on or against the patient may be avoided.

The ball syringe can also be employed in conjunction with
a good-sized gum elastic catheter (No. 12), and a small piece

of tubing, with very efficient results. In this case the catheter, after being well oiled, should be passed up the rectum, which can be done to a further extent than would ever be safe with the nozzle of any enema syringe; the short piece of tube attached to the other end of the catheter must then be joined to the nozzle of the ball syringe. The enema, having been carefully measured, can then be carefully and slowly injected, and all risk of its being drawn back into the ball syringe can be obviated by pressing the tube firmly with the fingers, and by pausing for a minute after all has been injected. The ball syringe can be gently detached before the catheter is removed.

Nutrient enemas are best given with the same appliance, and in the same slow, gentle way. The quantity should not exceed three ounces, and the object in both cases is to get the injection to be retained.

Eggs, strong beef-tea, usually peptonized, cream, with sometimes brandy and laudanum, according to orders, are the materials found best for the purpose, the object being to concentrate as much nourishment as possible into the smallest compass. They are more likely to be retained if the beef-tea is slightly thickened with a little arrowroot or starch.

Before administering nutrient enemas the nurse should ascertain that the bowel is ready to receive them, and not loaded with fæces. Nutrient enemas are usually ordered to be repeated at intervals, and there is no reason against making more than enough for one, at one time, provided you do not allow the mixture to get sour.

I think this concludes all I have to say to you in reference to a nurse's duty in connection with the administration of drugs.

LECTURE IX.

I HAVE frequently told you that careful, accurate observation is a very important part of a nurse's duty, and that the knowledge of how to use and cultivate that faculty is an essential part of a nurse's training. Doctors are often the first to admit the great assistance which you can be to them in this way, partly from the greater opportunity which being in constant attendance upon the patient gives you, and partly because women are universally acknowledged to have, for the most part, a natural gift for minute observation of detail which especially fits them for this office. Men frequently overlook what a woman of quite average intelligence will not fail to notice. You may decide for yourselves whether the masculine mind is too great for the reception of trifles, or whether it simply lacks this gift of quick perception, and leaves women in the superior possession of this quality! At any rate, you must *have* the faculty, if you are ever to make nurses; and now we will consider how you are to train and use it.

First, then, you observe for the purpose of reporting with absolute accuracy whatever may have taken place between the doctor's visits. Now for this reporting, remember, as the golden rule for your guidance, that it is your business to "state facts, not opinions." You must not enlarge upon what you have to say, and give long explanations. If you give the facts, fully, clearly, and concisely, the doctor can draw

his own conclusions, and it is not your business to draw them
for him, nor to state what your conclusions are. Be careful
never to give an opinion unless you are asked for it, and even
if you are under the impression that other treatment would
be better, or would have been tried by another doctor, it is
not for you to show that you think this either by word or
manner. Be *very* careful in your manner of speaking of the
doctors before the patients, and never give them *your* opinion
of their case as distinct from the doctors'. You must not be
afraid to speak, if it is your business to answer the doctor,
and so fail to give a truthful impression of what has taken
place. On the other hand, you need not fear exceeding your
duty if you keep to this rule of stating facts only.

Of course, if the doctor has been summoned for any urgent
symptoms, you will state at once for what he has been fetched.
If it is a regular visit, you will wait and first answer his
questions, and give as much information as you can in answer
to his questions, and *after* that inform him briefly and clearly
of everything else he ought to know. So much for the
manner in which you are to make use of your observation.
Now, in what way are you to observe ?

You must learn to observe on a system, not in a haphazard
sort of way. You must remember that hospitals are especially
places for the observation of disease. It is in these institutions that medical knowledge is made, so to speak. The
patients are placed under favourable conditions for those
skilled in such matters to be able to trace the course of
disease and the effect of remedies in a manner that can
scarcely be done to the same advantage under any other
circumstances. Therefore, if you are an experienced observer,
and a perfectly accurate and truthful reporter, you do not
need me to point out the *use* that it is in your power to be.

Nurses should use their senses in due order, and mentally
record what these senses teach them. Sight, touch, smell,

M

hearing, have all to be trained to do their duty from a nursing point of view. Experience will teach you the extreme value of all of them. Every careful night nurse will tell you how quickly she can detect a change—in the breathing of any of her patients, for instance; and I need scarcely point out of what vital importance the quick observation of such changes may be. Doctors aid these senses with the microscope, the clinical thermometer, the stethoscope, and many other appliances; but, of course, nurses can ascertain all that it comes within their province to know, without the aid of these things.

When patients enter the ward you will notice the *way they walk* or move, whether it is with difficulty, or easily; the extent of their helplessness, if it exists; their *colour and general complexion*, whether livid or pallid; the *pupils of their eyes*, whether they are contracted or dilated, whether they are of the same size; whether there are any injuries, and of what nature they appear to be; whether they complain of pain, and exactly where it is, and remember to quote the patient's exact words in describing pain; whether the breathing is of a normal character, or of what character it is; whether the patient swallows without difficulty; whether and exactly how long the patient sleeps, the kind of sleep, whether restless, heavy, or light; whether the motions and urine are passed in a natural manner, or unconsciously, and of what character these are; whether there are any twitchings or convulsions, and also as to the patient's mental condition, whether he is tranquil and apparently comfortable, whether he is indifferent to his surroundings or unconscious of them; whether in a state of stupor, of wandering, of quiet or active delirium. You will not need to comment upon *all* these points, but you should always notice them, in addition, of course, to the special symptoms of the disease from which he is said to be suffering. I should recommend you to practise the habit of getting these points into your mind about general cases where the information is not specially necessary. The habit will be invaluable to yourself always, and often of service to your patient.

You can ascertain by your sense of touch the comparative heat and cold of your patient. You will know whether the skin is dry and burning, whether it is moist and hot, whether it is cold and clammy, whether it is cool, or warm and comfortable. Notice whether the feet and hands are cold or hot. You can ascertain the actual temperature of the body exactly by the careful use of the clinical thermometer. I say "careful" use, for temperatures taken in the careless way I have seen them done, are worse than none. A wrong or doubtful temperature is more misleading than no record at all.

Many doctors are reluctant to admit that nurses are capable of taking the temperature of the patient; some are unjust enough to say that they never "trust a nurse's temperature;" but though this is a sweeping and probably an inaccurate statement, I must say that nurses are in a great measure to blame for the unsatisfactory impression which sometimes prevails on the subject.

Since clinical thermometers have come into such general use the Fahrenheit scale of measurement is almost entirely in use in England, so we will confine our attention to that.

The normal temperature of the surface of the body in health is marked on Fahrenheit thermometers at 98·4°, but there is also a difference of normal temperature in equally healthy individuals, so the extremes of temperature in health may be said to be from 97° to 99·6°. In health the temperature varies according to the time. It is normally lowest at two or three a.m., and highest about four p.m. It is most important to observe the greatest punctuality in taking temperature at fixed hours.

Doctors vary in their preference as to where the temperature shall be taken. Some prefer the axilla, others the mouth, and for children the rectum, and for some obstetric cases, orders are given for it to be taken in the vagina.

You must remember that the surface temperature averages one degree lower than the others, so you must not take it sometimes in one place and then in another, because that would be misleading as to the actual variation that had taken place. If, for any good reason, you are obliged to make the change, always note the fact distinctly. There is a little care necessary for getting a true temperature in the axilla, not only in noticing that the axilla is quite dry, and in removing any clothes from contact with the bulb of the thermometer, but in placing it so that the bulb is surrounded by and actually touching the body. It will not do this (as any of you can easily see if you try it on yourselves) by simply putting the arm under which you have placed the thermometer down by the side. You must bring it as far as possible across the body *in front*, and *if* you can make the patient hold the elbow of that arm in that position you will ensure an accurate result. *Never* let patients put in the clinical thermometer or take it out for themselves. I am afraid, or rather, I *know* that there are nurses who do permit patients to do both. How *can* you be sure that the thermometer has been properly placed if you let them put it in, and how *can* you be positive that it has not slipped if you do not take it out ?

I have spoken to you before about the importance of being very faithful over little things. I do not say that you will never have your temperatures doubted if they are carefully taken, but it rests with you never to have any doubt yourselves as to the perfect truth of the temperature you have ascertained. Every nurse who proves herself untrustworthy in these points not only creates a want of confidence in herself, but does harm to nurses generally, for often people do not pause to particularize when they have grounds on which to base a general statement.

A temperature taken in the axilla in the manner I have described can be accurately ascertained in five minutes, but eight or ten minutes is the time usually preferred.

In taking the temperature in the mouth the bulb of the thermometer must be placed under the tongue, and the patient instructed to keep the lips closed. Of course if the patient opens his lips and lets in the cold air you will not get the right temperature. You must also take care that the thermometer is placed *under* the tongue and not over it, otherwise closing the lips will not ensure the true temperature, because the cold air drawn in through the nostrils will come straight down on to the thermometer, and so prevent the mercury rising, or, at any rate, prevent its registering the true temperature of the patient. You may place the thermometer at the back of cheek or gums, if desired, instead of under the tongue. Three minutes is long enough to obtain a true temperature in the mouth, rectum, or vagina. I need not give you further particulars as to the manner of taking it in the last-named localities except to remind you to *oil* the thermometer.

Certain diseases have characteristic odours which experience alone can render familiar to you. Vomiting is a symptom that a nurse must report and notice. She must also be extremely careful about saving the vomited matter according to orders, and about keeping it covered, particularly from an infectious case. You can only learn from careful observation and experience in the wards, the character of motions, but you must always notice the colour, whether they are formed, solid, or liquid, whether they contain undigested food, worms, any streaks of blood or pus. If you observe anything abnormal you should always save them for some

one more experienced than yourself to see, whether you have
had orders to that effect or not. Be most particular about
saving motions when you have orders to do so. Neglect in
this respect is thoughtless and inefficient. You must always
be able to inform the doctor whether the patient's bowels
have acted, and how many times.

You will frequently have to save specimens of urine for
testing, as most of you know. You must be scrupulously
careful as to the cleanliness of the vessel into which the
urine is passed, and in which it is saved for inspection. It
should be kept covered to prevent dust getting into it. If
you notice anything abnormal you should save it for the
sister to see, even if you have had no special instructions to
do so. The dark inky appearance indicating that it contains
carbolic acid may be passed over unknown if a nurse, who
may be the only one who has a *chance* of noticing it, is careless enough to throw it away. It may be interesting to you
to know as broad facts that urine passed after taking food is
the most acid, and that while digestion is going on it becomes
almost alkaline. With animal diet there is less acidity, with
vegetable diet there is an excess of acid.

Acid urine turns *blue* litmus paper *red;* alkaline urine
turns *red* litmus paper *blue.*

The normal quantity of urine passed in twenty-four hours
is about fifty ounces. Nurses are frequently required to
measure the quantity of urine passed in the twenty-four
hours, and to take the specific gravity, so you should all avail
yourselves of the first opportunity of becoming acquainted
with the use of the urinometer. You must remember that
this measurement in the same way as degrees on the thermometer, is a purely arbitrary statement. It has been
settled that the specific gravity of water should be measured
by a definite figure of 1000, and that this should be taken as
the starting-point, so to speak; and with this acknowledged

this scale of measurement conveys a definite and universally the *same* idea.

The specific gravity of healthy urine varies from 1015 to 1025. Below 1015, albumen is usually looked for; above 1025, sugar.

In certain circumstances the urine may contain albumen, sugar, bile, blood, and pus, and other substances, and it will be interesting to you by-and-by to know what are the different tests for ascertaining whether, and in what proportion, the urine contains either of these things. But I must leave this to be explained to you later on, and content myself with merely drawing your attention to the fact.

Nurses must notice also if there is anything abnormal in the manner in which the urine is passed; if there is retention or any pain and difficulty; if with stoppages at intervals, as frequently happens with "stone cases;" if there is incontinence of urine. Most of you know enough physiology to understand that the lungs, the skin, and the kidneys are the three chief means by which impurities are removed from the system, and, therefore, that any defective action on the part of one or other of these organs throws additional labour on the others, consequently you can quite realize the importance of attending to any of these symptoms.

You will be expected to give an account of the patients' appetite—whether they take their food at all, whether eagerly or reluctantly, whether they retain it, and how much; whether they are thirsty, whether they complain of nausea, or whether they actually vomit. Then you must be very particular to get into the habit of speaking definitely as to quantity, and to be as nearly accurate as you can. Do not say "this patient took a good dinner;" "this patient has not eaten much," but try to say exactly, or as nearly as you can guess, what he actually has taken by weight. For instance, so many ounces of meat or fish, so many ounces of bread or

potatoes, so many ounces or pints of liquid in such and
such a time. Those are *facts*, and will be concise information
for the doctor's benefit, whereas the vague statements so
frequently given are of comparatively little use.

As different sorts of food are needed by us to supply various
physiological requirements, there is a distinct object in helping
the doctor with clear information as to what has or has not
been taken. Without attempting to enter fully into that
subject, that will be brought in detail before you in the final
course of lectures, we may just pause to think what an
important part of a nurse's duty the efficient administration
of food is. Food is absolutely essential to keep the body
going in a condition of health. It is needed to keep up heat,
muscular and brain power. If a person is starved, he loses
weight, vitality, the capability of doing work, physical or
mental, and the temperature falls. The body kept without
food is in somewhat the same condition as a fire kept with a
scanty supply of fuel.

Now, when people are ill, food is even more essential;
but it is necessary that the nourishment be supplied to
them in such a form as to render it of use to them in the
condition in which they are. It must be both digestible and
nutritious. Food to be of use must be brought into such a
condition that it can be absorbed into the blood, that is,
"digested." When the body is weak and ill, food in a form
that could be taken in health is of no service, because it cannot
be used. For instance, there are conditions in which a solid
piece of meat would wholly fail to convey nourishment, and
be worse than useless for that purpose; but if the nutrition it
contains be used in the form of beef tea, it will be of service,
because it will not only be nutritious, but digestible, *i.e.*
brought into such a condition that it could be absorbed by
the blood. Food, to be nutritious, must be digestible; but all
things that are digestible are not nutritious. The object of

cooking is to increase the digestibility of substances. Sometimes, as we well know, this object is defeated by the ignorant and inefficient manner in which cooking is done. Of course without cooking it would be impossible to get nourishment of many kinds into a convenient form for administration, such as mutton broth, beef tea, etc. Cooking also changes the condition of food; in a raw or cooked potato, for instance, there is a difference both in nutrition and digestibility. Then, not only the form, but the kind of food is of great importance under the varied conditions of disease.

You can readily understand that an alteration of diet or a refusal to alter it may be based on reasons that you cannot always see or follow, and consequently trained nurses must be slow to attribute to caprice any little incidents of the kind which may come under their notice. There is great scope for your skill and ingenuity in the way of preparing and administering diet. When you have the diet ordered, much depends upon you as to whether it is taken by the patient or not. Exquisite cleanliness; no dripping from the glass, cup, or spoon, as the case may be; nothing spilt in the saucer; bringing it fresh to the patient, and not leaving it for him to see and smell until he turns against it altogether; taking care that, if it is intended to be served hot, it *is* hot, and not lukewarm; not running off to fetch a knife or fork, or some other trifle that you ought to have thought of, such as salt, for instance, when the patient is waiting. *All* these are points which depend upon *you*, and your failure in any of these details may be the sole cause for the patient refusing what otherwise he might have been persuaded to take.

Punctuality in administering nourishment of every kind is most important. You should ascertain the doctor's wishes on the subject of waking your patient to give him food. In some cases patients would sink from exhaustion if allowed to sleep on without it, and for others undisturbed sleep is of

infinitely greater service. Patients frequently sleep better
after taking nourishment. A draught of warm milk or beef
tea will sometimes soothe patients off to sleep when they have
been wakeful for hours. A quiet, skilful nurse, that a patient
has grown to feel a restful confidence in, will often be able to
rouse her patient sufficiently for him to drink the required
nourishment without completely waking him up, and this is
one of the many occasions on which a gentle manner and
quiet movements are such invaluable qualifications for a
nurse.

This is the best system on which to observe, from a
nursing point of view, that I can recommend to you. Now
that I have put it before you, I can only hope that you will
all make it your business to carefully cultivate this habit of
intelligent observation in yourselves.

There is one other subject that I must not pass over
without comment in these lectures. I mean the last duty
which falls to a nurse's share when the life of her patient is
over. It is a sad, and often a very disagreeable task, and it
needs all the refinement and reverence of which you are
capable to do it as it should be done. It is the one thing that
each one of us will inevitably need done for ourselves, and let
us take care that we do, in each instance, as we would be
done by in this respect. The less talking that there is of any
kind the better; and loud, noisy talking there must be none.
Remember the impression any coarse, unfeeling, or frivolous
remarks must make upon the other patients ; and, while you
must endeavour to be quite bright and cheerful with *them*,
and not let the sad occurrence in an adjoining bed depress
your other patients or throw a gloom over the ward, there
is all the difference between that and letting them feel that
you are "hardened" to it. Do not forget what keen observers
and judges of character many of your patients are. Do
not hurry unnecessarily. Some of you, who are witnessing

death-beds for the first time, have probably been startled by
a sudden expiration of air from the lungs some time after all
breathing has ceased, though this does not always occur.
When all is over, the body should be laid flat, pillow and
clothes removed, the limbs straightened; the jaw should
be tied up by a bandage, with a slit made to take in the
chin, in order to afford firm support, and place the mouth
in as lifelike a manner as possible; and this should not
be removed until sufficient time has elapsed to ensure its
being firmly set. Take great care that the eyes are firmly
closed. They will often remain so if you keep your fingers
on the lids a minute or two; but if there is any further
difficulty, a pad of wet lint, pressed firmly across, will
generally accomplish it, or two-shilling pieces, though that is
not quite so nice. It gives a most distressing and ghastly
appearance if this point is not carefully attended to. It is
best, if possible, to remove the garments immediately before
any stiffening sets in; but it is not always possible to do this
if the friends are near, and you must be guided by circumstances.

After leaving the body for a little while, usually about an
hour, it must be washed. Keep it as decently covered during
this process, as though it were conscious the while; close the
orifices with cotton wool, if the nature of the illness renders it
necessary—you know there is often a great deal of discharge
after death; put on a night-dress—it is more convenient if
it fastens down the back; and lastly, if sufficient time has
elapsed, remove the bandage from the face and arrange the
hair smoothly. For the sake of the mourners you should
make the face look as much as possible as it did in life; if
there are any wounds let them be bandaged up with cotton
wool or lint. In some hospitals the bandage is not removed
from the head and face until after the body is taken from
the wards. When the men come to fetch it away, a nurse

should always stay by to assist them, whether there is anything actually for her to do or not.

Most earnestly I implore you not to allow yourselves to forget the solemnity of the office which you are called upon to perform—one death, two deaths, in a night or day, is the business-like and not unnatural way of speaking of the heavy amount of work which occasionally falls to your share; but do not let familiarity induce or excuse irreverence. Probably *your* hands are giving the last touches to those that have been dearly loved by some one no longer near—then treat their dead as you would have yours treated if it were not your privilege to be near them. And if it is a sadder case still, where no friends exist, where it is difficult to believe that any one ever can have loved the poor degraded man or woman whose miserable life of sin has closed in utter loneliness in the wards of a hospital, surely you will be pitiful and courteous in every touch, remembering the promise, "Whatsoever thing thou doest, to the least of mine and lowest, that thou doest unto Me;"* and that thought, too, will help you to bear patiently and without complaint the most revolting physical part of your task. It *does* call for self-denial; all I would ask of you is to exercise this self-denial freely. You will not forget that of old this work of showing reverence to the dead fell much to the share of women, and in endeavouring to overcome your very natural horror of some of these details, would it not be well for you to reflect that this piece of your work demands all the delicacy and womanliness which you possess, or which you can possibly cultivate? I confess that I sometimes tremble for the deteriorating and hardening effect which the frequent repetition of these scenes of sorrow and suffering has a tendency to produce upon you, particularly upon the youngest and most thoughtless of you; but do let me urge upon you who are

* Longfellow's "Legend Beautiful."

beginning, now while I have the opportunity, to be on your guard against this influence, and never let yourselves tend upon a death-bed, or be in the presence of the dead either in the hospital or elsewhere, without recognizing "that the place whereon thou standest *is* holy ground."

If you do this you will find, as life goes on, your character will strengthen, your sympathies will deepen with your fuller experience, and instead of growing harder and narrower and untouched with the feeling of others' infirmities, you will have the blessing of realizing that it has been very good for you to be there.

LECTURE X.

I SHOULD not consider these lectures complete, even in the very limited sense in which I intend them to be so, without devoting one to the subject of sick children. The nursing of children is a speciality, and requires special training and study. It needs infinitely more knowledge, more skill, more observation, and more patience to become a really good children's nurse, than it does to attain an average amount of efficiency as a nurse for adult patients. Indeed a moment's reflection will serve to convince you of this, if you have not fully realized it before.

It is essential for you to recognize the enormous difference that exists between the characters and dispositions of adults and of children. You will remember the familiar words, " When I was a child, I *spake* as a child, I *understood* as a child, I *thought* as a child." This statement is true of each one of us, and, in one sense at any rate, it is true that we have now " put away childish things."

When you enter a children's ward, you encounter a world in itself, of which the inhabitants are " little people," with different language, different manners, different feelings, different thoughts; and to nurse these little patients well it is necessary to understand them. Before you can do this you will have to study them very carefully. You all know the difficulty of nursing some of the poor foreigners that are brought to us. " It is so awkward," you naturally exclaim;

"he doesn't speak one word of English, and I cannot half make out what he wants." But the case of the little ones with a nurse who is ignorant of their ways is even more distressing, for the reasoning power of an adult at least places more means at their command of conveying their ideas to you, whereas the children under such circumstances are helpless indeed. Many of you are familiar with the following quotation from George Eliot's writing :—" Children, like the birds and beasts, have often an overflowing abundance of language, but it is language which is wholly inadequate to express the blind longings and aspirations, the wounded ambitions, the moral perplexities, the hungry craving for boundless love, with which many a sensitive child is burdened. In this deepest sense childhood is always more or less dumb, even when most noisy and talkative. He who would understand a child must not only listen for his words, which indeed are often somewhat futile, but must learn to read the unwritten speech of eyes and hands, and feel and watch with observant sympathy, not only the tears and smiles, but the gay caresses and appealing gestures and quick blushes, which it is possible to ignore or misinterpret."

There are many reasons why you should all endeavour to become very " understanding " in your dealings with children —besides the desire to become proficient in every branch of your profession, with which I trust you are all animated. Many of you who perhaps feel but slight interest in children now, will probably be mothers yourselves by-and-by, and then how thankful you will be for the knowledge that you now have such splendid opportunities for acquiring. In short, few women can go through life without finding themselves in circumstances which make them bitterly deplore their ignorance of the ways and needs of children, or deeply grateful for every item of knowledge which they may possess concerning them.

Maternal instincts are very real, very true, very beautiful —I would not say one word that could be interpreted slightingly of them—but you may be very sure that they will not supply or take the place of definite information concerning the proper treatment of children ; one day or night in the children's ward would suffice to convince you of this. How many out of the whole number of cases in the wards at any one time have been qualified for admission by the lamentable ignorance, not to speak of the neglect, of those to whom they belong ? If you take a newspaper and make a casual calculation, you will see that in the monthly average of deaths half of those that die are children under five—one-half of the whole total. Imagine what a terrible proportion ! Again, it has been calculated that one child in every five dies within a year of its birth, and that one child in every three dies before the age of five. These are sad and serious facts, and I want you to recognize their importance, for it is the plain duty of women, and therefore still more of nurses, to interest themselves in all that concerns the welfare of children. To you is entrusted the task of guarding the lives of the little ones from the beginning, and you who are constantly coming in contact with such pitiable little specimens of humanity, scarcely need me to point out to you the disease and suffering and misery which may result from ignorant or neglectful treatment in childhood, and the ruined lives of those men and women who have been the unhappy victims of such neglect.

Now, children differ markedly from adults in their physiological condition. They are *growing*, and that means a great deal. Their course of life and growth may be, and often is, interfered with by external circumstances, and imperfections of various kinds are set up in the growing child which cannot afterwards be remedied. This is mainly the case with the imperfect diet so frequently given in infancy and childhood. The bent legs so often occurring in children, from the weight of the body being too great for the legs to support it, is another fact incidental to the growing condition of the patient. An adult, however disproportionate the weight of his body might be, would not get bowed legs in consequence.

It is also noteworthy that the *vitality* of children is greater. They often can resist injurious influences that would be fatal to an old person, though, of course, there are certain diseases especially characteristic of infancy and childhood. Diseases in children run extremely rapid courses, and in many cases you will find that the child has either improved or passed away in an almost incredibly short space of time. On the one hand you will notice that they struggle through illnesses that would apparently be fatal to an adult, and on the other hand you will observe that the thread which binds a child to life is very slender, and will break almost before you have time to realize that there is any danger of it.

Now, if we admit that the organs of children are in a distinctly different physiological condition from those of adults, it is not difficult to understand why nourishment must be supplied to them in such a form as to enable them to make use of it. I have already told you that all food, to be nutritious, must be digestible; and it follows, therefore, that we have to take great pains with the diet of children to ensure its being of such a kind and administered in such a form as can conveniently be disposed of by the child's digestive organs. Injudicious feeding is the cause of a large proportion of the diseases of infants. Deplorable ignorance prevails, more especially among the mothers in the class of life from which most of our patients come, as to the kind, the quantity, and the regularity of the feeding necessary for them.

Children should, during the first few weeks of their lives, be fed about eight or nine times in the twenty-four hours, and as the child grows to be a few months old this number

N

should be reduced to about four or five times in the twenty-
four hours, and you should be careful to accustom the child
to take its nourishment regularly. Infants suffer exceedingly
from flatulency, and this suffering is materially increased
either by over-feeding or too frequent feeding, or from keeping it too long without food. I need scarcely point out to you
the folly of supplying a child with food every time it cries,
as some mothers and nurses get into the habit of doing. Probably the baby is crying from pain which a fresh quantity of
food may only increase, whereas gentle rubbing of the child's
abdomen would frequently soothe the little creature, and
help to dispel its constant source of discomfort, wind. Of
course children *do* cry because they are hungry—crying is
their chief means of making their wants known—but it is
absurd to imagine that children are always hungry because
they cry.

If you have to bring up an infant " by hand," as it is
called, you may like to know that the quantity of milk considered desirable is, for the second day, about a quarter of
a pint. The first day it scarcely takes anything. By " day "
I mean in this case the twenty-four hours. The third day
it takes about two-thirds of a pint, the fourth and fifth
day about one pint, and from this it gradually increases, so
that by the time the child is six months old it is usually
taking about two pints of milk in the twenty-four hours.

Cow's milk, diluted with one-third of water, is usually
suitable; but there is no universal law on the subject. You
must note whether the milk you are giving seems too heavy
for the child in question. It may be that if you mix it with
equal parts of barley water and slightly sweeten it, the child
will be able to digest it readily, or by adding more water
than usual, or some lime water, may possibly be the best
means of adapting the food to the requirements of any particular child. Sometimes cow's milk does not do at all, and

then other kinds must be tried. The condensed Swiss milk
diluted with two-thirds of water is generally found very
satisfactory.   There are innumerable " foods for infants "
recommended and sold in all directions, but the drawback in
nearly every one of them is that they contain *starch*—a
material that very young children are physiologically unable
to digest, so that these foods are not only useless, but, in
different degrees, positively harmful to the little creatures
who are the unhappy victims of your ignorance if you insist
upon feeding them with it.

The appearance of the first teeth is nature's indication
that other food besides milk may be given with advantage—
boiled bread beaten up in the milk, Robb's biscuits, and
possibly by this time a little arrowroot may be given. But
remember, these additions must be introduced very slowly
and in very small quantities. Do not forget that the fact of
a child taking what you give it is not the slightest proof of
its being good for it, as many mothers thoughtlessly imagine.
I wonder how often you and I have heard, in answer to the
doctor's question of " How do you feed it ? " the well-known
answer, " It has a bit of what we has ourselves," and further
inquiries will elicit the fact that probably a bit of bacon, of
meat or fish, or plum-pudding, for instance, forms a part of
the unwholesome diet cheerfully given by these well-meaning
mothers to the poor little creatures entrusted to their care.
We must not blame them for ignorance which perhaps they
have never had a chance of remedying, but if you as nurses
will bear in mind the statement I have just made to you as
to the wholly different physiological condition of a young
growing child to that of a full-grown adult, you will at once
understand how it is that children fed in the manner now
described may be positively starving for the want of the kind
of food that could be digested by them, the sort supplied
being worse than useless for providing nourishment to organs

that are not as yet in a sufficiently developed state to receive them.

Mothers will understand that they would be badly nourished if kept on the sort of food given to infants, even if supplied in large quantities; and you should endeavour to make them see that in exactly the same way infants are starved on the kind of diet which seems satisfactory to them.

Feeding-bottles require constant attention from the nurse, and whenever possible two should be kept in use for one child, to be given alternately, and the one not in use, after careful cleansing, should be kept in clean water until you want to use it again. The bottle itself can be cleaned like any other glass without much trouble. A little raw potato chopped fine, or a little shot shaken up in it occasionally, will clean and brighten it very effectually; but it is the india-rubber part of this feeding apparatus which is a constant source of difficulty; it so frequently and quickly becomes sour. If the child declines its bottle your first thought should always be, is *any* part of it sour? Remember, it must be absolutely sweet and clean. Do not examine it carelessly, and after a hurried glance or smell say to yourselves, " There is not much wrong with it; it will do for this once." If there is anything wrong with it, it will not do at all! The best way to ensure and maintain a perfectly cleanly condition of this india-rubber tubing is to remove it from the bottle directly the infant has finished its meal, and wash it thoroughly before the food has time to dry on it and become sour. Of the two, it is easier to prevent its getting into a sour condition than to get it nice again when it has become sour. Please recollect that this is one of the most important points a nurse has to attend to in the feeding of infants. Weaning under ordinary circumstances should take place at the age of nine months, though there is a great deal of variety on this point, for many reasons.

I said that the appearance of the first tooth indicated a certain stage in the child's development, and it may interest you to know one or two particulars concerning the teeth.

The first set with which nature supplies us are called milk teeth, and are twenty in number, ten in each jaw. The second set, which replace these later on, and are called permanent teeth, number thirty-two, sixteen in each jaw. The first teeth we expect are the two central incisors—usually these appear in the sixth or seventh month; two lateral incisors, about the eighth or ninth month; two canines do not appear until about the eighteenth month; but two molars appear from the ninth to the twelfth month, and the other two molars about the twenty-fourth month.

After five years children generally begin to lose these teeth, and they are gradually replaced by the permanent set. Most children suffer a good deal during teething, and are very fretful and restless with the pain. Convulsions are not infrequently brought on at this period. This is always rather an anxious time for those who have the care of babies; but you may remember, as a general rule, though there are exceptions, that they do not take measles and other diseases more or less incidental to childhood until after they have reached their first or second year.

It may be a matter of passing interest to you to know that the average weight at birth of a male infant is estimated to be seven pounds eleven ounces; of a female infant, seven pounds four ounces. This reminds me to beg you to be most careful in weighing such cases as you are instructed to weigh with every care; accuracy is of great importance to the doctor.

I have spoken of the feeding of children first, because it is closely connected with the point of the physiological difference between a child and an adult, and I am anxious to impress this fact upon you; but I scarcely know if I am right in

letting cleanliness take the second place.   At any rate, let me
beg of you not to regard it as a secondary consideration.   I
am not afraid that you will exaggerate the importance of it,
for that is simply impossible.   Not only would many forms
of skin disease be far less rife if scrupulous cleanliness were
insisted upon, but no drugs, nor even good feeding and pure
air, can supply the place of it.   Children *must* have clean
bodies if you mean them to be healthy, and, though you may
smile at the notion, I can assure you that keeping them clean
materially assists them to be good.   You may always observe
how happy a healthy baby will look after it has been made
clean and comfortable, whether it has enjoyed the washing
process or not, and a great deal depends upon the way the
ablutions are done as to whether the child takes the per-
formance placidly.   Whenever possible, a morning bath,
given at about the same temperature as the child's body, is
very desirable.   Let it be rapidly done, and the child
thoroughly dried and wrapped up to prevent chill.

   Some children are frightened at the mere idea of a bath;
but this is generally the result of bad management.   As a
great part of the good to be derived from a bath would be
prevented by any shock or fright, this should be patiently
guarded against, and the child be gently encouraged to like
it.   Occasionally the sight of the water terrifies the child,
and then it is best to cover the bath with a blanket, and let
the child gradually into the water by putting it on the top,
and letting it sink into the bath by degrees.   By this means
a timid child will grow half-interested in watching the water
come through the blanket, and be spared all alarm at the
process.   It indicates tact and good management on the part
of a nurse when the little children under her charge enjoy
their baths, and I am inclined to think that the contrary
qualities are suggested when the reverse is the case.

   However, the sick or injured children, that *you* have

mainly to consider, cannot often be treated in this manner, and so you must wash them thoroughly in bed, though it takes a little longer, and gives you more trouble. After you have thoroughly washed and dried their backs, dust them freely with starch or zinc powder. You cannot take too much pains to prevent a chafed and abraded skin. And once more I must take the opportunity of reiterating my warning against the dirty habit of washing more than one child in the same water. The idea is sufficiently repugnant in connection with a healthy person, need I point out to you how much the objection is intensified in sickness ? I do not for one moment do you the injustice to suppose that you would deliberately run a risk of infection to any of the patients entrusted to you ; but what I do want you to see is that it is your business to think of and understand these things, and that if harm is done through ignorance or carelessness on your part, it cannot be excused on these grounds. A separate towel, separate flannel or piece of lint, and separate water for each patient should be a rule without an exception in a children's ward.

I need scarcely point out to you the necessity of changing draw-sheets and napkins directly they are soiled. It is your one chance of avoiding sores and of keeping the atmosphere of your ward fresh and pleasant. It is often difficult, even when you have done your best, always to have them fit for the doctor's inspection in this particular. I can only say, *do* your best, and always have them as nice as you possibly can for your own satisfaction.

Many of the children have been badly educated in habits of cleanliness, and you may do a great deal for them, and save yourself trouble by judicious management. It is an excellent plan to place those who are able on the necessary utensil early in the morning and after each meal. Persevere with this, even if you do not meet with success at first. Usually after children wake up from a sleep this need should be anticipated. Encourage them to call for what they want, and praise and recognize their little efforts to be good in this respect. This method will obviate the necessity of scolding, and be of more service.

Children are very troublesome; there is no denying the fact. Their little wants are endless; and when you have many under your care, all crying and wanting things at once, the most devoted lover of children may be forgiven for *feeling* wearied and impatient with them, though not, perhaps, for *showing* it. The self-control which some nurses exhibit under worrying circumstances is truly admirable, and cannot be too cordially emulated by others who are anxious to excel with children.

Keep the body-linen of the children frequently changed and aired. I have already pointed out the advisability of changing the night-dresses of those who are living in bed every night and morning when possible.

It is very troublesome sometimes to keep the splints of children in a clean condition, especially the padding. There are so many difficulties in the way. Cover them with oiled cotton as much as possible, to keep any moisture from soaking through. On the other hand, you have no idea how rapidly lice generate in splint pads, especially when assisted by this covering of oiled cotton; so look out carefully for them, and be sure and tell the sister at once of the first suspicion that they have begun. Plaster of Paris splints and others of that description are best varnished over after the splint has dried, so as to render them impenetrable to moisture. A coat of spirit varnish is the best and safest application you can use. Box splints are quite a comfort to a nurse in helping to maintain cleanliness, because they enable her to turn the little patient round on its face, and clean and relieve the constrained position without risk of too much movement to the injured limb.

The third essential to the well-being of children, after suitable diet and cleanliness, is plenty of warmth, light, and fresh air. Warmth is a necessity for children. If they are deprived of it to any great extent, they *die*. It is, unfortunately, no unheard-of thing for cold to be the active agent in killing some of the poor neglected little creatures in our overcrowded cities. A certain amount of external warmth is essential, and children do not possess sufficient vitality to dispense with it. I mean that, in proportion, children are infinitely more sensitive to cold than adults. Acute chest attacks are far more fatal to children than to grown-up people.

Then children cannot flourish without *light*. It is the want of light and fresh air which stunts their growth, and has no small share in producing the pallid little objects with which our London streets abound. We do not expect the flowers to grow without sunshine, nor the trees to bring forth their foliage, neither can the very colours of the insect be developed without light; and as we have learnt this from observation, we may well take the hint that nature aids us with, and give the children as much light and sunshine as there is to be had from the first thing in the morning to the last thing at night. Children rejoice in light by instinct. Who, that has noticed a child at all, has not seen how its eyes will follow a lamp or a candle about, or how it will lie steadily and blissfully blinking at it? Poets and moralists have had a great deal to say about the child's efforts to grasp at sunbeams, and most of us have smiled at such a sight. Perhaps it would be as well for us if we did not grow so very unobservant of the sunbeams as we grow older. However, I have said enough for you to know the importance of this detail. I need not add more than a passing comment upon the necessity of giving children fresh, pure air when they are asleep, because I have already made you fully aware of the

importance of it; but I mention it as a distinct fact for you
to keep in remembrance.

I shall not say very much to you about the different
diseases of children, because we have already spoken of many
of them under other headings. Tracheotomy is one of the
most anxious cases through which you can nurse a child.
This operation and the nursing of it we have already discussed
in detail.

I have also told you of the extreme care necessary in
moving cases of hip disease, but I remind you of it now,
because it is chiefly with children that you have to do with
it. *Do* be careful to keep the limb perfectly straight when
you raise the child, and the head rather lower, if anything,
than the rest of the body, to prevent any additional weight on
the inflamed joint; stand on the well side, with the diseased
or injured limb *farthest from you.* Any jerk is perfect agony
to the unhappy victim of this complaint, so pray be very
careful not to swing the weights to and fro when you are
dusting the cot, or to knock up against them when you are
hurrying up and down the ward. When you have to move
the cot in which such a patient is, do so slowly and steadily,
not with a sudden push. If the disease is at all advanced,
those upon night duty will find that the patient is apt to wake
up from a deep sleep with a shriek of pain—a cry indeed
which is in itself characteristic of the disease to those who are
familiar with it; sometimes they scream thus in their sleep,
but more often they wake up in a fright. This cry is due
to the spasm of the muscle which pulls the two inflamed
surfaces of the diseased joint violently together, causing in-
conceivable agony. Always go to the child, and see that the
weights are all right, and the limb in good position; and,
above all, never scold it for making a noise, as though it could
help it. Persons suffering from hip disease nearly always
complain of pain in the knee, instead of in the hip itself. You

will perhaps wonder that I lay so much stress upon the
nursing of this one class of cases ; but if you had spent as
many nights and days as I have in the wards of the Alexandra
Hip Disease Hospital, and had opportunities of seeing how
very much the suffering of these patients is increased or
diminished exactly in proportion to the ignorance or skill of
the nurse, you would not wonder that I am so earnest in
beseeching you to be tender with these children, and to give
yourselves the trouble of learning how to handle them.   It is
so pitiful to see a little thing sobbing for half an hour with
the torture it has to endure through the clumsy touch of a
well-meaning person, who, *if* she is a nurse, remember, ought
to know better.

Cases of burns and scalds I have already spoken of, and
the careful manner in which they must be undressed when
they are carried into the ward—that is, if they are in a condition to be undressed at all.   Children, with their sensitive
organization, bear shock very badly, and many, many cases
are fatal from this cause.   The various applications used, the
manner of applying them, and the importance of keeping a
burnt or scalded surface covered up from the air, are matters
on which we have previously spoken.

There are still a few points to which I must call your
attention, but having done that, I must leave you to make
the practical observation which alone can render these hints
of any service for yourselves.   Study the faces, the expression,
the colour of sick children.

A celebrated French physician, who had charge of the
hospital for "waifs and strays" in Paris, stated that he
was able to diagnose children's diseases from the lines and
furrows on their faces.   I tell you this, not for you to do the
same, but to show you how real such indications must be, and
to show you, too, how thoroughly worth while it is for you to
study the signs written so clearly for those who " have eyes

to see." Without entering into the more obscure details which follow the statement of this distinguished man, you may remember this : That with pain in the head you generally find contraction of the brows; with pain in the chest the nostrils stand out sharply and work rapidly ; with pain in the abdomen you may generally notice a drawing-in of the upper lip.

There is a good deal to be learnt from the colour. Lividity of the lips and eyelids shows a weak condition of the circulation ; a faint purple tint of the eyelids and round the mouth indicates some difficulty in digestion. A general earthy tinge of the complexion is a sign of chronic bowel complaint. These are broad general statements which could be multiplied a hundredfold were it necessary for our purpose.

The *cry* of a sick child varies in a most curious manner, and conveys much information to those skilful in the interpretation of these sounds. In brain disease you get a sharp, short, sudden cry. If the child is crying from stomach-ache, the cry is more prolonged and wailing ; if a child is hungry, thirsty, or suffering from ear-ache, it will cry almost without ceasing, because the cause is constant and does not occur in paroxysms. If the child is suffering from inflammation of the chest or windpipe the cry will naturally be hoarse or whispering. I might describe these signs to any extent, but I have said enough to show you the many directions in which you, must seek the valuable amount of information that an intelligent observer cannot fail to discover.

I have not yet said anything about providing amusement for children, but it will not be wholly disregarded by one of their special nurses. As a matter of fact children have a marvellous capacity for amusing themselves, if they are well enough to be amused at all. You cannot have toys scattered all over the place when you are expecting the surgeon, of course, and, as a rule, children are very amenable to judicious

management, and much influenced by each other's example,
either in the way of being good or being naughty. But
while order is good, and neatness indispensable, I should
like to see a little more tact exercised occasionally in the way
of a wise exception to this rule, such as giving a doll, or a
toy, or a book, to a little new child whose grief at finding
itself amongst strangers would be gradually mitigated by
this arrangement. There have been occasions on which I
have had reason to fear that some of you are not as careful in
soothing the little ones, when they are first brought to us, as
you might be with advantage. *We* know that they will be
perfectly happy again in an hour's time, but *they* do not know
that, and it is just that point which makes all the difference.
Children live, in the present, they do not look forward or
backward—this is universally a characteristic of childhood.
Try and realize this ; it will help you much in your en-
deavours to understand children. Victor Hugo, who has
depicted some of the most tragic scenes which have ever
happened in this world, and painted the miseries that men
and women suffer in powerful colours, says positively that
there is no misery like the misery of children. And this is perfectly true, for the joys and sorrows of childhood fill their
whole minds and hearts. They are quite as intense as they
are transient, and I cannot say more than that. Children's
brains, children's ideas, children's thoughts and ways, are not,
as a rule, sufficiently studied. We do not half recognize the
struggle that the tiny creature goes through. How it strives
to grasp matters far beyond its reach, and puzzles its little
brains to comprehend what goes on around it, and beyond.
It is a great mistake to suppose that children do not think.
It is true they do not think and reason *as* we do, but they
understand more than we have any conception of. The faith
and trust of childhood is one of the most beautiful things
that we ever get the chance of seeing. It is our own fault

if we shut our eyes to it. In our turn we have much to learn from the children. If we could have retained our belief in truth and the splendid realities of life and nature, as we felt them in our childhood, do you not think that in many respects our daily lives would be grander, nobler, and higher than they are? and in this sense we should do well to take a lesson from the little ones and remind ourselves that " of such is the kingdom of heaven."

And this brings me to a matter that I must not pass over in silence—I mean the use that you should make of having these untaught, uncared-for little ones brought under your influence from the squalid life of sin and misery outside our walls. They come in to be nursed—yes, that is true, but that is not all. Dozens of these little ones may never have another chance of learning what it is in your power to teach them, and that, too, without any extraordinary expenditure of time and effort on your part. You are kind to them, and you have all experienced how readily children respond to love, and how sweet it is to see their little faces brighten up at the sight of you. They tax your patience, but I think when I sometimes see the contented way in which these little mortals are nestling themselves in nurses' arms that you have your reward. What chance have the children of comprehending what love means when they see no ray of it penetrating their daily surroundings? They learn to curse as soon as they can speak, just as readily as they would learn to pray if they had had the chance, for children are naturally imitative. At whose door does the result lie? Let them leave the hospital with fresh thoughts in their young minds. It is your part to sow the seed, and be cheered with the thought that good seed cannot fail to bear fruit, though you may never see it. You may not only be the means of helping the child, but that child may have opportunities, which never could have been at your disposal, of showing light to others.

George Eliot encourages us with a beautiful thought on this subject : " In old days there were angels who came and took men by the hand and led them away from the city of Destruction.   We see no white-winged angels now.   But yet men are led away from threatening destruction ; a hand is put into theirs which leads them forth gently towards a calm and bright land, so that they look no more backward ; and the hand may be a little child's."

In conclusion, then, think no time wasted that is bestowed upon the children.   Be gentle and good to them for their sake and for your own.   It would be a very old, weary world, if there were no children in it to keep us fresh and hopeful.   I imagine that we shall all be inclined to admit the truth of another of George Eliot's wise sayings : " We should never have loved the earth so well, if we had had no childhood in it."

LECTURE XI.

The nursing of fever cases and questions of infection and disinfection, as far as these matters come within a nurse's province, are subjects full of interest to all of us.

You seldom have the nursing of so-called infectious diseases in a general hospital, as they are very properly removed to institutions set apart for them; but there is always the chance that you may have them to attend to. Those of you who are preparing for private nursing are almost certain to have a good proportion of them, inasmuch as every one is more or less liable to be the victim of infection. The importance of your thoroughly understanding all the duties which fall to a nurse's share in connection with these illnesses is increased by the fact that in this kind of nursing you have not only the welfare of your patient to consider, but the welfare of the public, in preventing the spread of such diseases, and also you have to guard your own health in every way possible, without, of course, making the comfort and wants of your patients a secondary consideration.

Those of you who are interested in general questions of health, apart from the details that come strictly under the heading of nursing, would do well to get yourselves a cheap little American book, entitled " Long Life and How to reach It," by Dr. Joseph Richardson. It contains a great deal of practical information, conveyed in very simple language, and amongst other subjects there is a chapter on " contagion, and how to escape it," which you might all spend ten minutes profitably in reading. One or two points I shall quote from it this evening.

Contagion means " to touch together," and " is the term applied to the material in consequence of which a healthy person, *touching* a diseased one, may have conveyed to him the disease with which the latter individual is affected. The word infection is applied to the substance or influence by which a malady is transmitted from one person to another, either with or without actual contact."

You will, therefore, understand that whereas all *infectious* complaints must be contagious, all contagious complaints are not necessarily infectious. Numerous and violent are the controversies which have been waged, and are still being carried on, in regard to the true nature of contagion. Probably there is no subject on which doctors are more at variance than this one. But it would be quite out of place for me to speak to you of any of these varied theories.

We have not to deal with the scientific side of the question, absorbingly full of interest as it is ; but the details of putting into practice such measures as have been accepted as serviceable more or less universally, or such as may be deemed desirable by the particular doctor for whom you may be nursing, it is our *duty* as far as possible to understand. It is distinctly from this point of view that I am anxious to put before you some definite information to-night. It is a great help to a nurse to be familiar with general rules for her guidance in any branch of her profession. It may not always be well or possible to follow them, but if variations from them are the exception, that does not detract from their value in the majority of instances. Knowledge is power in everything, and in the case of trained nurses intrusted with the charge of patients suffering from diseases ready to spread to innumerable victims if you will let it, *what* power the judicious

o

exercise of this practical knowledge of yours places in your hands! One of the greatest blessings we are ever granted is the opportunity of helping others; one of the greatest pleasures is the conviction that we really have been of service, and this is a pleasure that you as nurses will often in future be able to secure if you take pains to duly qualify yourselves.

Knowledge of the general laws of health and for the prevention of the spread of disease cannot be too generally diffused. Do not lose sight of this fact, for many will be your opportunities of giving information to those who are thankfully leaving their friends and relatives during these infectious illnesses in your more skilful hands. The majority of people take but passing, if any interest at all in these matters, until some person they know happens to be the sufferer. Then, when their personal interest is awakened, they will be eager to learn all the practical information on the subject that you can supply them with, and they will naturally look to you for it. Take care that you have it ready to bestow upon them, otherwise there will be another means of good left undone through ignorance.

I have recently been reading rather an interesting lecture on preventable diseases and their causes, delivered by Dr. Smart at Edinburgh some two or three years ago. He describes a preventable disease as "one which arises or spreads in consequence of the wilful, careless, or ignorant violation of those laws, the proper observance of which we know to be necessary to insure the preservation of health and avert the spread of disease. . . . Accepting, as we do, the theory that each case of infectious disease originates in the reception of a distinctly specific, pre-existing poison, and that it in turn becomes self-propagating, we will first point out some features which are common to the whole group, and then speak a little in detail of the distinctive characteristics of each of these 'zymotic diseases,' as they are usually called. They all begin with a period of what is termed either 'dormancy' or 'latency,' or more generally 'incubation,' during which the poison is actively developing. But the duration of this period differs in each disease, and there is considerable variety in individual cases in each disease. These differences in the length of the incubation period are probably due in each instance to the amount and strength of the poison received.

"These fevers are all ushered in by a marked and sometimes sudden elevation of temperature, which, with variations, continues during the course of the illness. It is because of this increased temperature that they are called fevers. Characteristic eruptions next appear." Unfortunately we have no remedy that is able either to cure these disorders or to shorten their duration; and we are obliged to content ourselves with placing the patient in the best hygienic condition, and with treating such complications as may present themselves as they arise.

Patients should be confined to bed during the whole course of the fever, and all bodily and mental exertion must be strictly prohibited. The room must be maintained at an equable temperature, not exceeding 60° Fahr., and plenty of fresh pure air must be admitted to the patient. Free ventilation is of the utmost importance; and all carpets, curtains, screens, and other furniture likely to interfere with this must be removed. The room must, of course, be kept quiet, and if the patient shows much tendency to mental excitement and delirium it will be best to darken it.

Patients suffering from fevers may generally partake freely of liquids, such as water, iced water, toast-and-water, barley water, and so on. Many of you may be familiar with the popular prejudice—which formerly existed to a much greater extent than it probably does now—against giving cold water to patients with fever, and greatly must the suffer-

ing of these unhappy victims, parched with thirst, have been
increased by this well-meaning but ignorant treatment. I
mention this because it is well for you as nurses to know
that there are no grounds for this prejudice. But remember
that these patients will be eager to drink all they can get,
and you should not put into their hands too large a quantity
at one time and expect them to drink a little of it. Put as
much as you intend them to have in the vessel they are to
drink from, and then give them a fresh supply when they
need it. They may have frequent draughts of water, but not
too much at one, time; and with children it is very thoughtless to make them cry by giving them a cup or a feeder full
of water and then to take it away from their eager little
lips when you think they have had enough.

Food cannot properly be digested when fever is running
high, so patients are usually kept without solids, and nourishment is supplied solely in the form of liquids. But of course
the doctor will order the diet he may prefer for each
individual case.

Another point which nurses can scarcely lay too much
stress upon is the necessity for absolute cleanliness, not only
of the patients' surroundings, but of the patients themselves.
There is a curious dread of washing and sponging patients
when they are suffering from these complaints. It is thought
that the rash would be "driven in" if the surface is touched
with water. This popular belief has probably arisen from
a well-founded horror of patients suffering from fever "getting
a chill," and very serious reason there is for extreme care in
guarding against such a possibility. Most of you already
know enough physiology to be able to form some idea of the
exceeding danger of checking the action of the skin at any
time, and this danger would be immensely increased in a
condition of fever. It would result in extra work being
suddenly thrown upon the kidneys, producing in all pro-

bability inflammation of those organs, followed by dropsy and other grave complications.

But you are well aware, as nurses, that there need not be the very slightest risk of taking cold either in frequent sponging or in frequent changes of linen, but that, on the contrary, the patient will be relieved and benefited by both. The passage of a damp sponge, not quite cold, unless specially ordered, is a source of great comfort to a patient whose skin is dry and burning with fever, and not only of comfort, but of positive service, as this tends to *increase* the action of the skin.

I think this serves to illustrate the value of good nursing. Here is a remedy and a means of relief which doctors dare not avail themselves of if they cannot rely upon its being skilfully administered, and I hope this fact will serve as an inducement to you to take pains about apparently trifling details. Carefully air the bed and body linen, but you need not insist upon putting it on warm, if it is not agreeable to the patient. The sensation of the cold linen against their burning limbs is generally very welcome to any one suffering all the discomforts of a high temperature.

Now let us speak briefly of the conditions under which infectious diseases are considered to spread.

The generally accepted theory is that infecting germs may be dispersed in a variety of ways—wafted by the air, carried by water and milk, or conveyed by our clothes, our money, or the innumerable commodities given in exchange for that. There can be little doubt that in the majority of cases the spreading of these diseases is brought about by the healthy coming in contact with the sick or convalescent. Children after these attacks are allowed to go back to school long before such a step can be taken with safety to their companions. Laundresses disseminate the poison amongst their employers, when the linen from these cases is sent them in an infected state; and these women, too, have lost their lives before now from receiving clothes that have come, impregnated with fever poison, straight from fever patients. I name this source of infection specially because it is one with which the nurse has much, or, indeed, everything, to do. There are numberless other ways by which each of these fevers can be conveyed, but I need not now dwell upon them at greater length. We can with more profit turn our attention to the details that nurses have within their own control. To begin with, let us take the regulations for nursing typhoid fever which the physicians of this hospital desired to have carried out in our wards. I commence with this— not that typhoid fever is infectious, in anything approaching the same degree as the other class of fevers, of which we will speak presently, but because it is the one which you have unrivalled opportunities for studying here.

Typhoid fever differs from all the others, in its being but slightly, if at all, infectious through the air; and it is for this reason that, with perfect safety to ourselves and the other patients, we can with certain precautions nurse it freely in our general wards.

This malady is generated by the contents of sewers and cesspools, and by the drinking of impure water or milk. The seat of the attack is the intestines chiefly, and the poison is mainly eliminated by that channel. It is accordingly the intestinal discharges that have to be most carefully looked to, and every precaution must be taken by disinfection and removal. These discharges acquire their maximum infective power when decomposing. Now suppose you have a case already diagnosed typhoid, when it is brought to the ward, in the first place remember that—

1. Patients' clothes are to be sent to the fumigator as soon as taken off.

2. All vessels (feeders, cups, jugs, bed-pans, etc.) in use

for the patient are to be marked and kept *entirely for that patient's use.*

3. All linen (sheets, shirts, etc.) is to be put into a metal pail (provided for the purpose) containing carbolic solution (1 to 19). If the linen should be soiled with evacuations, the pail is to be brought to the bedside, so as to avoid carrying such linen through the ward, and infecting by their effluvia.

4. Before giving bed-pan or urine-bottle to patient, put some carbolic solution in it; and, after use, cleanse with carbolic solution. (Bed-pans must *always* be carried covered.)

5. No discharges from the patient are to be left under the bed. They must be taken away at once, and, if to be reserved, put (with carbolic solution) into a glass pan in the lavatory—such pan to be covered.

6. Sprinkle under and round the bed constantly with carbolic solution.

7. A basin of water containing carbolic solution is to be kept near the patient's bedside, into which the nurses are recommended to dip their hands after attending to the patient's requirements.

8. Cleanse the thermometer in carbolic solution after each time of using.

I may tell you, though it does not come within your province to see after it here, that boiling is the surest way of disinfecting contaminated clothing, or baking in an oven heated to about 240° Fahr. But remember, if you ever attempt disinfecting linen by the boiling process, the germs will only be destroyed by water at boiling point. That kills them, but any warmth short of that makes them grow; so be very careful.

These directions are so clear that I think I need make no comment upon them, or pause to impress upon you the importance of conscientiously carrying them out. Any failure of duty on your part may be indirectly, or perhaps directly, the cause of fatal results to yourself or others, and I hope this reflection will have due weight with you.

There is one other point that I may as well mention now, because it is well for a nurse to remember it, in addition to these, for other fevers, though it is superfluous as a precaution against typhoid. I mean the desirability of hanging up a sheet soaked in some disinfecting solution, and particularly placing one in the form of a curtain over the door that may lead into uninfected parts of a house.

If the air is impregnated with poisonous germs, it is a very reasonable theory to load the atmosphere as far as possible with the antidote to that poison; and remember that, if employed at all, the sheet must be kept thoroughly saturated with the disinfectant, otherwise it will be of no service. It is for this reason that, when you suspect the occurrence of an infectious case in the wards, you immediately surround the bed with clothes wrung out in carbolic acid solution or some other disinfectant, to prevent the germs that may be emanating from the patient filling the atmosphere of the ward. You should also remember to use a damp duster in the neighbourhood of an infectious case, and not send the dust, which may be mingled with poisonous germs, flying about in all directions.

The special characteristic of typhoid fever is ulceration of a particular portion of the intestines. This is the main cause of the tenderness of the abdomen on pressure, and this is the chief reason why you have to keep your patients absolutely at rest, not allowing them to sit up, and not allowing them to stand or get out of bed on any pretext whatever. This also explains why it is a matter of such vital importance to keep these patients without solid food of any description. When you conceive the risk of perforation of the bowel, which may so easily ensue if any hard article of diet comes in contact with, or gets deposited on, membranes in this condition of ulceration, I think you will be more than ever careful with these patients yourselves, and consider no trouble wasted in impressing upon them and their friends the great necessity for enforcing to the letter the doctor's orders concerning liquid diet.

In typhoid fever the bowels are relaxed, and the motions of a light ochre colour. Sometimes they may contain blood, and this is a most important symptom, and must be carefully watched for.

Frequently a number of rose-coloured spots appear upon the abdomen and elsewhere, and these vanish on pressure, and return when the pressure is removed. Each one lasts about three days, and then fades insensibly into the hue of the neighbouring skin, and other spots follow. Sir Thomas Watson tells us that these spots begin to show themselves, generally, during the second week of the disease, and fresh spots come out every day or two till the third week, in the course of which they cease to appear, except in cases of relapse, when they also may recur with the other symptoms. This eruption of rose-coloured spots in successive crops is highly diagnostic of typhoid fever. Sir William Jenner holds that this species of fever is over by the thirtieth day, since, under ordinary circumstances, no fresh spots are seen after that day. Of course the *illness* may continue much longer, protracted by the effects of the fever, or by pre-existing local complications. Dr. Murchison states that the pupils of the eyes are dilated in typhoid fever.

You must be exceedingly careful and accurate in taking the temperature of these cases. It is a symptom full of interest to the doctor, and one which may be actively guiding his treatment. Any sudden drop of temperature must be carefully noted, and promptly reported. It may possibly be the result of drugs given to lower the temperature, or it may be the first indication of internal hemorrhage or other serious symptoms. I mention this, as some of you might be apt to imagine, from the fact that so much attention is paid to bringing the temperature down, that the decrease must of necessity be satisfactory. It *may* be, and, on the other hand, it may be quite the reverse; so pay great attention to this and corresponding symptoms.

Complete recovery from typhoid can never be announced till the evening temperature shows perfect freedom from fever.

Sometimes slight epistaxis, *i.e.* bleeding from the nose, occurs in typhoid fever; but it is not a serious symptom, unless the bleeding is profuse.

You will, of course, be careful to have the patient placed on a spring bed, with a hair mattress and light bedding.

The patient must be kept in a recumbent position, but not lying on the back, as he often has a great inclination to do. He must be very gently turned partially round from side to side, and supported in that position by pillows carefully arranged for the purpose. This is done partly with a view to preventing the occurrence of bed-sores, and partly to obviate the tendency to pneumonia.

Typhoid patients should never be allowed to sit up, except when it is essential for the doctor to examine them, and then they must be very carefully raised and supported. In certain stages of typhoid fever the act of sitting up suddenly might induce perforation of the bowel, and syncope —I mean sudden failure of the heart's action—has always to be guarded against in these cases. The nurse must not forget to notice the quantity of urine passed by a patient suffering from typhoid fever, nor fail to report the fact if there has been any temporary retention.

I think this is all I need say with regard to the *general* nursing of typhoid fever. All special treatment you will be

very careful to carry out intelligently and carefully, and remember that each physician will have his own view as to the
desirability of bathing, sponging, cradling, and so on, and the
nurse's part is implicit obedience to those views in every case.

Typhus fever is highly infectious, and you are not likely
to see much of it in a general hospital. Nevertheless, it is
desirable that you should be told something about it. It
is said to be "caused by overcrowding and deficient ventilation, and it is very apt to attack those who are exposed to it
for the first time." The poison is thrown off by the skin
and lungs, and readily infects the atmosphere, clothing, and
furniture, so that the chief precautions are those of ventilation
and disinfection.

Sometimes typhus fever sets in suddenly with a rigor
and a temperature of about 104° Fahr. the first evening. The
thirst in typhus fever is usually troublesome for the first few
days. Delirium does not come on as a rule till towards the
end of the first week. The muscular power is greatly
depressed sometimes, even during the first stage of the dis-
order, the prostration is extreme, and the tendency to stupor
and indifference to surrounding objects very great. Towards
the end of the first week the eruption peculiar to typhus
fever commonly begins to show itself, though sometimes it
does not appear until later. Sir William Jenner calls the
eruption which is distinctive of typhus fever, "the mulberry
rash." After the third day of the eruption no fresh spots
appear. It disappears in the course of the third week of the
disease. The character of this rash varies with its age. It
is never papular, but consists at first of very slightly elevated
spots, of a dull crimson colour. Each spot is flattened on its
surface, irregular in outline, and disappears completely under
the pressure of one's finger. In two or three days these spots
undergo a marked change. They are no longer elevated, they
become darker, dingier, more defined, and then they only *fade*

and do not disappear under pressure. From this condition the
spots in most instances grow paler, pass into faintly marked
reddish-brown stains, and finally vanish. The spots or stains
composing this mulberry rash are generally very numerous,
set closely together, and sometimes they almost cover the
skin. They are usually spread over the trunk and extremities,
occasionally over the trunk only, and now and then they are
seen on the face. Each spot remains visible until the whole
rash disappears. To this rule there is one exception. The
eruption sometimes shows itself first on the backs of the
hands, and leaves those parts within twenty-four hours.
When numerous the spots have not all the same depth of
colour, consequently the surface has a mottled look. It is in
the course of the second week of the disease that death is
most apt to take place in typhus fever.

Typhus fever, after the first week, has a characteristic
odour of its own, by which nurses learn to know it. Dr.
Murchison suggests that the vapour which imparts this
smell, imparts with it the typhus poison, and he tells us also
that the pupils of the eyes are usually contracted in typhus.
During the third week of typhus fever, the patient's chance
of recovery improves. When convalescence has once fairly
begun it goes on rapidly, and recovery from typhus fever is
mostly both early and complete.

This disease is much less fatal to young children than it
is to adults; after fifty-five years of age it is said to destroy
one-half of those whom it attacks.

Now, with regard to small-pox, or variola. Dr. Smart
tells us that there is no contagion so strong and sure, or that
operates at so great a distance, passing from house to house
and from street to street. The patient charges the air, and
everything about him, with a most subtle and deadly virus,
derived chiefly from the skin, and mucous membranes, but
not restricted to them.

As you all know, the only protection against this terrible disease is vaccination, which should be repeated at least once after the fourteenth year.

Dr. Richardson observes that " people of the present day, who complain of the temporary inconvenience and almost infinitesimal danger of vaccination, can only do so through ignorance of the horrible suffering, disgusting deformity, and appalling mortality which attended small-pox in former times. It is estimated that in England during the eighteenth century, nearly one-third of all the inhabitants, ladies included, were pitted with small-pox, which caused about ten per cent. of all the deaths taking place every year. The mortality was so great, that one out of every four, and, in some epidemics, one out of every three, attacked, died of this frightful malady; and when we remember that every one seized with it became immediately an object of danger, dread, and loathing to his best friends and nearest relations, and, if he or she recovered, was generally rendered repulsive-looking for life, we can faintly realize what a blessing Jenner's discovery has been to the world."

Small-pox usually sets in with sharp, feverish symptoms, rigors, followed by heat and dryness of skin, with nausea, vomiting, and pain in the back. Children do not shiver, you know, so in their case it is sometimes ushered in with an attack of convulsions, which is the equivalent to a rigor in an adult. The peculiar eruption almost always begins to show itself on the third day of the fever. At first the pimples feel hard like small shot under the skin. The earlier it comes, the more severe the attack is likely to be. The eruption comes out first on the face, then on the neck and wrists and on the trunk, and lastly on the lower extremities. As a rule, it does not cease to come out until the fifth day. " The severity of the disease is almost always in direct proportion to the quantity of the eruption. The number of pustules

indicates, in the first place, the quantity of the variolous
poison which has been reproduced in the blood.   In the
second place, it is also a direct measure of the extent to which
the skin suffers inflammation.   Sometimes there are not more
than half a dozen pustules; sometimes there are thousands.
If all these were collected into one, it would be an enormous
abscess.   For both these reasons the system suffers commo-
tion, distress, and peril in proportion to the quantity of the
eruption."   When the pustules are very many they run
together, and then it is called "confluent small-pox."   The
pimples gradually increase in magnitude, but it is not till the
third day of their appearance that they begin to contain a
little fluid on their summits.   It is the eighth day of the
disease, and the fifth day of the eruption, before they become
perfectly turgid.   During the time in which they are thus
filling up, the face swells; often to so great a degree that the
eyelids are closed and the skin between the pustules on the face
assumes a damask red colour.   About the eighth day of the
eruption a dark spot makes its appearance on the top of each
turgid pustule, and at that spot the cuticle breaks, a portion
of the matter oozes out, and the pustule dries into a scab.
This process begins on the face, and pursues the same course,
only two or three days later, upon the extremities.   The feet
and hands swell just as the face swelled, but they begin to
swell just as the features begin to resume their normal
size.

Many things are recommended to relieve the intolerable
itching and to prevent the pitting which is so frightfully dis-
figuring.   Painting the surface with collodion, castor oil,
nitrate of silver, carbolic oil, glycerine, vaseline, and so on;
but of course you will always use the application ordered, and
nothing has as yet been discovered to be infallible for this
purpose.   There is least risk of fatal termination between the
ages of ten and fifteen; below five the complaint is often fatal,

and after forty the danger increases in proportion to the age of the patient.

Chicken-pox is a very trifling complaint, and seldom requires much treatment beyond a warm bath. It generally begins with slight fever, and within twenty-four hours a number of small reddish pimples appear, generally on the back; the second day these become vesicular, and by the fifth day they have generally disappeared.

Measles begin with all the symptoms of a common cold, running at the eyes and nose, sneezing, hoarseness, cough, and difficulty of breathing; the characteristic eruption usually appears on the fourth day. It is two or three days in coming out, beginning on the face, neck, and arms, then reaching the trunk, and finally the lower extremities. " In this course it resembles the eruption of small-pox. It fades in the same order, standing out for three days at least upon the face, before it begins to decline; so that its whole duration comprises a space of six or seven days. It becomes browner as it fades. You may feel that the eruption is slightly elevated above the general surface of the skin, especially upon the face, which is somewhat bloated and swollen. The parts which the rash has recently occupied are left covered with a dry, small seurf, which crumbles away in a fine, branny powder. You may remember that, unlike small-pox, measles are not severe nor dangerous because the eruption is plentiful and early. The eruption is the distinguishing feature of measles, but the catarrhal affection is in every way the most important. Diarrhœa is very apt to set in when the rash is fading, but the great danger of measles is pneumonia, which is very likely to supervene. The period of incubation for measles is from ten days to a fortnight. The contagion is active enough, but certainly it is less strong and diffusive than that of small-pox.

You should use soft pieces of old rag or linen, instead of

good pocket handkerchiefs, to wipe the eyes, mouth, and nose of patients suffering from measles, as these discharges are highly infectious, and it is best, when possible, to burn material that has been in contact with them.

Scarlet fever is generally marked by the characteristic affection of the throat and the distinctive rash. It is highly contagious, and much more to be dreaded than measles. The period of incubation for scarlet fever is short, usually not exceeding five or six days, sometimes briefer still. The rash of scarlet fever commences in minute points, which speedily become so numerous and crowded, that the surface appears to be universally red. "They begin on the neck, face, and breast, and extend to the extremities, pervading at last every part of the skin. It is peculiarly distinct at the bends of the joints and on the chest and abdomen. The eruption usually stands out for three or four days and then begins to fade, disappearing altogether, as a rule, towards the end of the seventh day." About this time desquamation of the cuticle begins to take place—in small scurf or scales from the face and body, in large flakes frequently from the extremities.

The best way to prevent infection from these particles which peel off is to anoint the patient all over with carbolic oil, and this should be continued from the fourth day for six weeks. If the patient is not able to bear carbolic oil, or the doctor does not approve, he may possibly allow olive oil or simple dressing to be rubbed over the patient's skin. Any process which is likely to prevent the infected skin flying about in a fine powder is very important, and, of course, if the cuticle can be disinfected before it comes away from the patient, so much the safer and better for all in contact with him. The patient cannot be considered safe to mix with others until the peeling is quite over. The severity of this disease is chiefly marked by the extent of the throat mischief;

the tonsils may be simply inflamed, or they may become the seat of extensive ulceration and even gangrene. You can hardly attach too much importance to the necessity of guard-ing your patient from all risk of cold during the convalescent stage, for the slightness of the attack of fever is no guarantee against the susceptibility to many diseases which scarlet fever leaves. Inflammation of the kidneys, Bright's disease, dropsy, are among the serious diseases to be feared as the consequence of any carelessness in this respect.

After the process of desquamation is entirely over, Dr. Richardson recommends that the patient should still be kept isolated for a week, and should have a daily bath containing carbolic acid solution, so that at last every square inch of the body will have been thoroughly disinfected. Be very careful, too, about the head and the hair, for the disease poison, both of scarlet fever and of small-pox, is apt to linger among the dandriff that accumulates at the roots of the hair.

Diphtheria, whooping-cough, mumps, are all highly in-fectious, but I think there is nothing special I need tell you about them in addition to what I have already said.

Now, in conclusion, there are two extremes that nurses must avoid with regard to infection as it concerns themselves —the cowardly dread of it on the one hand, and the careless disregard of it on the other. Perhaps you will think it strange that it is the latter extreme that I am most afraid of for you; but I am sure that is the one which is the more likely to prove a temptation, unless you are carefully on your guard against it. Women who fear infection for themselves are greatly to be pitied; but they have no business to be nurses, and the sooner they understand that they have mis-taken their vocation the better it will be for themselves and all concerned. Many unselfish people may fail as nurses from lack of other essential qualities, but you may be sure that no woman lacking *that* qualification has any fitness for

P

the work at all. Except perhaps a natural shrinking that
may come across the bravest of you as the possibility of your
catching some horrible disease suggests itself to you, there
are not many nurses who find the idea a difficulty to them;
neither must you suppose that I regard it as a selfish thing
to have the sensation of fear. It is not wrong or anything
but natural to have such a feeling occasionally; the wrong
would only be in allowing one's self to yield to it.

If our wards were filled with an epidemic of cholera or
plague to-morrow, instead of our regular cases, I have not
the slightest doubt that nearly all of you would be as eager
to nurse them as though it were not fraught with great
danger to yourselves. But when it comes to the other extreme
of taking infinite pains and trouble to guard against the
infection that you have ceased to fear in the slightest degree
yourself, and with which you are so familiar that you have,
to all intents and purposes, ceased to realize its existence,
then many of you are not so conscientious in putting into
practice the knowledge you possess; indeed, it is not too
much to say that many experienced nurses are culpably
negligent in this way. We are all apt to forget or to ignore
what we do not see or feel, and to take but little definite
notice of our everyday surroundings, and so perhaps there is
nothing so very remarkable in the fact that this generally
accepted attribute of human nature should be painfully
illustrated by nurses who devote their time solely to the care
of these cases. If only infection were a visible instead of an
invisible danger, and if only it could be borne in mind that it
is as real as though it could be felt and seen and touched,
what a comfort and help it would be!

What I want to impress upon you is that nurses *know*
the importance of taking these precautions which have
been enjoined upon them. Probably they have done their
best conscientiously to carry them out to the letter, until

familiarity has made them careless and indifferent. Now,
do you honestly think that any nurse has a right to
excuse herself, or to expect others to excuse her, for the
neglect of a single detail, when she *knows* the consequences
may be so terrible to others ? And, after all, the carelessness
of which I speak seldom arises from anything but sheer
laziness—or, I fear I should add, a want of *trustworthiness*.
Perhaps you may not do any harm. That is true. But,
then, how can *you*, who *know* what you are doing, run the
risk ? The mischief done may never be traced home to you,
but does that alter the case ? Let me implore you again to
be very faithful over the little things ; or, if you cannot make
up your mind to all the trouble that entails, give up nursing
the sick, and find employment that does not bring the health
and happiness, and perhaps the lives, of your fellow-creatures
into your hands. I speak and feel forcibly on this matter.
It is no exaggeration to say that it is one which involves
questions of life and death to others, and of the carrying out
of high principles as opposed to lax and slovenly work from
yourselves.

The great encouragement in nursing fever cases is that so
much depends upon the nursing, as far as the result of the
disease is concerned. All nurses have a weakness for patients
who "do them credit," and it is the feeling that you are
fighting a stern battle, the issue of which depends largely
upon your care and skill, that so animates nurses with hope,
and rewards them for the anxiety of their work.

There is always the *possibility*—it is not more than that,
for the proportion of nurses who "catch" things from their
patients is very small in the aggregate—but there *is* the
possibility which no nurse need shut her eyes to, that she
may have to suffer herself, or that she may meet her death
as a direct consequence of attending to her patient. I have
already spoken to you of the quiet courage that nurses need

to possess, and the possibility of danger to herself makes no
true woman turn from a clear call of duty. It is only natural
that I should anxiously hope that none of you will be called
upon to suffer in this way; but if it does happen that the
angel of death thus greets any one of you, you will never
regret that he found you at your post, using your nurse's
talent faithfully to the end. The highest things that are
worth living for are worth dying for too, if the need arises;
and if you are in earnest you will not be afraid that any
good to others will cost yourselves too dear. "Let love be
your motive and reward while you live." That is the
truest and the most encouraging thought that I can ask you
to take for your guidance in this, and indeed in every branch
of your work.

LECTURE XII.

To-NIGHT I propose to say a few words to you in reference to the ventilation, temperature, and light of your wards or sick-rooms. I have not left it until the last because I consider it of minor importance, but because there were other details more likely to be of interest to probationers on their first entrance into hospital life.

Dr. Anderson, in his admirable little book on " Medical Nursing," says—" Air may be regarded as invisible, without colour, taste, or smell. . . . It is not a simple body; it is not one of the elements, as the ancients supposed, but a compound body. It consists mainly of two elements, oxygen and nitrogen. Oxygen is a gas, without colour, taste, or smell; it sustains animal life, and supports combustion, i.e. it enables fuel to burn. It is the life-giving principle of the air, although there is only one part of it to four of nitrogen. Nitrogen is also devoid of colour, taste, or smell. It extinguishes life and light. It modifies the vital properties of the oxygen, or, as has been said, ' it dilutes the oxygen as water does wine or spirits.' These two elements form almost the whole bulk of the atmosphere; but there is a third body, which, although there is only a trace of it in the air as a whole, is so poisonous in itself, and so readily increases in circumstances that concern us very directly, that we must give it our most careful attention. I mean, of course, carbonic acid gas. This is a compound body devoid of colour, but with a slight smell, and a rather sour taste. It extinguishes light, and if breathed undiluted, destroys life instantly. . . . We cannot remain in a room without increasing the quantity of this poisonous gas. With every expiration we give out at once impure air—air so far unfit to be breathed again by our own selves. Hence arises the necessity for ventilation. But besides breathing out this poisonous gas, we continually remove some of the life-giving oxygen; the carbonic acid expired being formed by the combination of oxygen with the carbon of our bodies."

It is noteworthy that whereas animals, ourselves included, use up oxygen and give out carbonic acid, plants do exactly the reverse—take in carbonic acid and give out oxygen. Thus the atmosphere of the external world is kept clear. But there is one point in connection with this fact that you must remember. During the night, i.e. in darkness, plants give out carbonic acid, consequently you must never allow growing flowers to remain in a sick-room during the night. There is no possible objection to them during the day; on the contrary, they do positive good, and help to purify the atmosphere. But of course your own common sense will tell you not to select flowers with a very strong smell, unless they chance to be a special favourite of your patient. Now, " proper ventilation," says Dr. Parke, " is clean air displacing foul air constantly and steadily, without chilling the patient." Miss Nightingale writes still more emphatically on the subject, and declares that " the very first rule of nursing, the first and the last thing upon which a nurse's attention must be fixed, the first essential to the patient, without which all the rest you can do for him is as nothing, with which I had almost said you may leave all the rest alone, is this—' to keep the air he breathes as pure as the external air without chilling him. . . . To have the air within as *pure* as the air without, it is not necessary, as often appear to be thought, to have it as *cold*.' " *

* Miss Florence Nightingale's " Notes on Nursing."

You have, most of you, been here long enough to notice the attention paid to keeping the wards fresh and free from smell, and can judge of the importance attached to this matter by the trouble and expense incurred in procuring various ventilating appliances to facilitate the removal of impure air and introduce as much fresh air as possible from outside. Neglect of these precautions in an institution of this sort would be followed by outbreaks of pyœmia, erysipelas, and other more or less preventable diseases.

Without in the least disparaging any scientific apparatus which assists in maintaining a pure atmosphere in the wards, it has been proved by experience that the most effectual method of ventilating within the nurse's control, is opening the windows a few inches *from the top*. Nothing entirely supersedes this plan, and it is one which cannot be wholly dispensed with. If you open the windows at the bottom you will get a draught, probably coming directly on the patient, and all the inmates of the room, and run the risk of giving them rheumatism, stiff necks, and general discomfort, and that, too, without fulfilling your object of thoroughly purifying the air.

It is all very well to throw up your windows at the bottom when the external air is so mild and pleasant that you can give your patients the benefit of it without risk of chilling them, or of too far lowering the temperature of the room, but it is of no use attempting to keep the atmosphere fresh by this plan. To quote Miss Nightingale again—"The air throughout a room is never changed by a draught in the lower part of the room, but it *is* changed by an open window in the upper part."

Ventilation, to be thorough, must be systematic, and is not to be supplied in jerks now and again, just when you happen to think of it. It is the frequent changes of temperature which do harm, the sudden alternations between hot and cold which must be carefully guarded against and prevented, and the fresh, *even* temperature that you must take so much pains to maintain.

I have greatly to impress upon nurses that ventilation is an important matter, to which they must give unremitting attention, and any neglect of which will go far to counteract the good effects of skilful nursing in other respects. A plan for admitting fresh air into a room where cold draughts have to be carefully guarded against was suggested by Mr. Hinckes Bird, some time ago. The suggestion is, that a piece of wood about three inches in depth, and made the exact width of the window frame, should be inserted underneath the lower sash, which should close down upon it. In this way the air must enter by the space between the sashes, which, of necessity, are open when the lower sash is raised. The plan is really excellent. A still better and simpler way in new buildings is to have the lower sill made three inches *higher* than usual, so that if the sash is lifted just less than that you have the same effect as if the wood were there, no trouble of putting in or taking out, and no draught.

It requires plenty of judgment and common sense to ventilate judiciously. You have to fight against the proverbial horror of fresh air peculiar to the class of people from which most of your patients come, and which is frequently shared in, to a large extent, by better educated people, who have not studied the subject sufficiently to have overcome the popular prejudice. I believe this prejudice is strengthened, or at any rate is much slower in dying out, because nurses who have grasped the notion that an abundant supply of fresh air is indispensable, frequently forget that cold and draught are discomforts, and sometimes dangers to which their patients must not be exposed.

If you allow your patients to be cold as a consequence of bestowing fresh air upon them, it is not wonderful that they will prefer being warm and so far comfortable to being thus clumsily ventilated, and remember that in some cases by chilling a patient you may cause fatal results.

Patients who are in bed can always be kept warm with blankets and hot bottles, and yet allowed to have the air they breathe as pure as though they were out of doors—at least this is possible in well-built wards and rooms, and it is always the nurse's duty to do the best her circumstances will permit to attain this object. You do not want to air your wards from inside the building, but from outside. You must not forget that "if windows are made to open, doors are made to shut." If there is any necessity to have the door opened for a time, shut the window for that time, and do not keep your patients shivering in the draught because "it won't be for long." That is no reason for making them take cold.

Close the windows near the patients when the doctor is sounding them, when they are washing, or in any way exposed; but do not let the ward get close by forgetting to open them afterwards. Be exceedingly careful not to have wounds dressed with the draught from an open window coming upon them, or you will run a great risk of causing erysipelas. You will notice in accident and surgical wards, that patients suffering from open wounds are generally placed in beds away from the windows, not because they do not require fresh air, but because in these cases all draughts have to be so studiously avoided.

In medical wards it is becoming more and more the custom to place patients suffering from chest complaints near open windows, with the intention that the air they breathe shall be fresh with as much oxygen as possible; but it is at least equally important that they should be shielded from the sudden draught of cold air, which brings on a distressing attack of coughing that could by a little thought have been spared them.

The special prejudice against night air is so absurd that I should scarcely have thought it necessary to speak of it, only I know that you will again and again have an objection urged against it by your patients, and it is best for you to have some distinct ideas on the subject. " What air *can* people breathe at night but night air ? " And surely the fresh night air from outside must be more wholesome than the night air inside, which has been inspired and sometimes re-inspired over and over again. In large towns the night air is often the purest to be had in the twenty-four hours ; and it is said that the air in London is never so good as after ten o'clock at night. Take every convenient opportunity which presents itself to disabuse your patients' minds of the erroneous views prevailing as to " night air." I hope you will take as much care of yourselves in this respect in your own bedrooms as you do of your patients in the wards.

Until you have experienced it, you have no idea of the difference it makes, if you have been sleeping in a room where a fresh current of air has been circulating freely, or if you have been sleeping in one where it has been carefully excluded, and you have been breathing the same atmosphere over and over again. " The expired air is deprived of from three to four parts of oxygen, is charged with this noxious gas—carbonic acid—and also with morbid particles from the lungs and blood; and, until it is freely diluted in the sur-rounding atmosphere, is deleterious to animal life. If confined within a space, the air becomes overladen with carbonic acid gas, and deprived of oxygen ; therefore, a correct balance between the supply of oxygen and the demand can only be maintained by admitting a supply of fresh air from the outside." If you have opened your windows at the top and insured this, you will find that it does not require half such an effort to get up when you wake, which, I am sure, is an important consideration to all nurses, and that the tendency to headache which every one feels after sleeping in a close room is to a great extent removed.

You will discover also that it is not only physically but mentally beneficial to avoid an impure atmosphere. When people are cross and irritably inclined to quarrel with themselves and everybody with whom they come in contact, it sounds somewhat ridiculous to suggest by way of a remedy that the window should be opened; but, if you try the experiment next time, you will probably find it effectual in removing the fundamental cause of the mischief.

At any rate, when you are tired, listless, and disinclined to exert yourselves, when you know no special reason why this should be the case, it is quite worth while to discover how far it is due to the air you have been breathing. So much is within our own control in these little matters which affect our health and comfort to so large an extent in everyday life, that it is a great pity not to understand them, or to neglect to carry them out.

If you are not quite sure whether the atmosphere of your room or ward is fresh, you can always settle the point by leaving it and entering it again; for you know that those coming into a close place are far more conscious of it than those who, by remaining in it, have gradually become accustomed to the atmosphere. It is a great mistake for a nurse to suppose that letting out the fire will improve the ventilation, for very much the contrary is the case. It will make a room *colder* to let out the fire, but not *fresher*—very far from it, as the escape of warm air creates continuous circulation of air in a room. Many nurses are so far from understanding this, that when I have had occasion to remark that their wards were close they have often said, "I will let the fire down," as though that would be sure to improve it, whereas it would simply make it worse. The broad rule for ventilating, with common sense modifications to adapt it to circumstances, is—

"make up the fire, open the windows *at the top*, and shut the door." If the weather renders a fire inadmissible, of course you will be careful to see that the chimney is open, and not allow it to be closed up on any pretext whatever. A lamp placed in the grate will ensure sufficient draught for purposes of ventilation.

Now with regard to the warmth of the atmosphere in which you are keeping your patients. It is scarcely less important than their food. The temperature of medical wards is generally considered best from 60° to 64° or 65° Fahr.; surgical wards not above 60° Fahr., and sometimes a degree or two below that. This is the rule to guide you when you receive no special instructions on the point, but surgeons differ on this as on other questions, and if you are told to do anything different, you can only obey orders.

Many nurses apparently forget when the thermometer is placed in the wards that it is meant for them to refer to, and that it would be helpful to them if they cultivated a habit of looking at it regularly. I should recommend all of you to adopt this little plan for yourselves. You know what creatures of habit we all are, and if you get into the way of watching the variations of temperature now while you have comparatively very little to do with it, it will cease to be a trouble to you, and you will not forget it when you are taking staff nurse's duty and are responsible for the figure at which the mercury of the thermometer stands in your wards.

Nurses should regularly look at the ward thermometer whenever they come on and whenever they go off duty, for their own satisfaction, besides referring to it if they are in any doubt as to the *warmth* of their ward. In addition to this, night nurses should notice it towards the dawn, when that peculiar chill which precedes or comes with the very early morning, and which must be already well known to many of you, will certainly make the temperature fall below the

required heat unless the nurse has wisely taken precautions
to make up her fire and guard against her patients feeling it.

The light of your wards is another matter which needs
a little attention. Except in those cases where light is painful
or prohibited—chiefly brain or ophthalmic cases—the more
light and sunshine you can get into your wards, the better it
will be for all concerned. Of course you will not allow a
patient to lie with the sunshine streaming into his eyes, but
do not forget that the sun will not remain in that position all
day, and that if it has been necessary to draw down the
blind, you must draw it up again afterwards. Dark rooms
are never fresh, however much air may be passing through
them, and dark corners are not healthy. You may notice
that any dark or shady corner will retain a disagreeable smell
even if there is plenty of air in the immediate neighbourhood,
long after it has disappeared from the rest of the room.
Sunshine is a necessity, physically as well as morally, and
it has a definite and powerful influence for good in many
ways. You must carefully regulate the artificial light also,
and remember that a gas-burner is said to consume as much
oxygen and gives out as much carbonic acid as four or five
men. Two candles or one good oil lamp are computed to
have the same effect upon the atmosphere as the presence
of one man.

Now, I think it may be a help to you if I endeavour to
recall briefly the chief points which I am anxious that you
should keep in remembrance, as the result of your attendance
on this course of lectures.

You will all have realized that there is a wide distinction
between the work of a doctor and the work of a nurse; that
there is a marked difference between the kind and degree of
knowledge necessary for each in their respective callings.
Doctors and nurses both aim at precisely the same object,
namely, the cure of the sick, or, at any rate, the alleviation

of their suffering; and this object can best be attained—or, indeed, can only be attained—by each keeping to their own line, with the sincere desire of affording mutual help.

You will have understood, also, that nothing can be more opposed to trained nursing than "amateur doctoring," so that the slightest approach to this objectionable form of quackery will, I trust, be impossible to all of you. Keep the clear idea in your minds that nurses find their place as active agents in carrying out a scientific system of treatment laid down by the doctor, and if you reflect upon all that involves, it is not possible to overrate the importance of your position, or to mistake its limits.

I have explained to you that treatment usually presents itself to us under one or more of the following aspects :—

First, to provide an antidote to any poison, and to remove all sources of harm. Secondly, to put patients under the most favourable condition for self-cure. Thirdly, to aid in treatment by drugs which experience or experiment have shown to be efficacious.

I told you that one form of treatment only might be employed, or that a combination of all three might be considered desirable; but you will find that *all* treatment can be classed under one or more of these heads. Time will not allow me to repeat illustrations of my meaning, but I hope you will at least remember the fact.

Therapeutics—*i.e.* treatment—consists in the application of natural agents, such as rest, cold, heat, and so on. We have already spoken in detail of these things, for it is under the second heading—*i.e.* that of "putting patients under the most favourable condition for self-cure"—that most of *your* work comes. We have seen that these remedial agents—as well, of course, as innumerable others which have not as yet been told you—can be applied either generally to the whole body, or locally to any part for which they may be prescribed.

You will try and remember the points I have mentioned in connection with ordinary and special bed-making, with the washing of helpless patients, and other matters involved in a nurse's duties when her patient has to be kept absolutely at "rest." We have said some little, too, on the padding of splints and of other appliances for providing "local rest." You will, I hope, be able to efficiently administer any of the general or local applications of cold, which I so minutely described to you; and, at any rate, I trust I said enough to convince you of the positively harmful effect of allowing an ice-bag to remain on when it has become a bag of warm water. If you recognize the importance of such details, I am confident that we shall not meet with any such evidences of careless nursing in our wards. The administration of such forms of dry or moist heat as may be ordered generally or locally is, of course, not less important. You will not fail to be accurate and careful in reference to the temperature at which these remedies are applied by you; and you will not forget that dry heat can be tolerated at a much higher temperature than moist. It is not possible nor necessary to repeat the items we have previously dwelt upon, but please keep the manner in which these remedial agents act clearly in your mind.

Cold and heat act, then, by modifying the supply of blood to the surface—by diminishing it, which is the effect produced by cold; by increasing it, which is the effect produced by heat. In addition to this alteration in the quantity of blood, there is an alteration of sensibility—i.e. diminished sensibility, as by cold, up to complete loss of sensation; increased sensibility, as by heat, up to scalding, with all the varied degrees of sensibility between these two extremes, such as the sensitiveness of the surface after poultices or fomentations, or the coolness of a part after the continual application of an evaporating lotion.

The main uses of these natural agents, then, are: (1) to modify amount of blood to surface; (2) to reduce temperature; (3) to increase temperature.

They act as cold-producers, by direct abstraction of heat from the surface, by conduction, and by evaporation. You know that if you put any cold substance close to a hot substance, the hot one will give up heat to the cooler body; that is what we mean by losing heat by conduction. Evaporation is the passage of a fluid into a gaseous state, and during the process of evaporation heat is used up, and a fall of temperature is produced. Again, these natural agents act as heat-producers by the direct application of a hot substance, or indirectly by diminishing evaporation and thus preventing the fall of temperature.

I merely touch upon these points now with a view of recalling the fuller explanation of them that I have previously endeavoured to give you, and in the hope of leaving a clear impression of these subjects on your mind.

I need say nothing to recall such details as I have mentioned in connection with your work in preparing for, attending to, and nursing operation and accident cases. These subjects will now be brought before you in a more interesting form, and the repetition of them will serve to remind you of any small points I have put before you. The same applies to the remarks I have made in reference to medical nursing. But in the mean time go on actively cultivating your powers of observation, for this is a matter you must attend to for yourselves. Observe on the system I pointed out to you the other night, enlist *all* your senses in the service of your patients, and cultivate, from a nursing point of view, your faculties of hearing, seeing, smelling, and touching. A certain amount of experience is essential before these senses can be fully trained; but I have no hesitation in saying that this is far more a matter of education than of time. You may be in a hospital twenty years, and leave it absolutely ignorant of the meaning of systematical observation of your patients, and rest under the delusion that you know your work, because from long habit you cannot fail to notice the existence of some striking symptom ! Whereas, in a very short time you may so have acquired the *habit* of methodical observation, that in every case you come across you will only have to turn your attention to the symptoms of that individual patient, and then none of them will escape you for want of your powers of perception having been trained. It is of no use taking up a book full of wisdom if you cannot read the language in which it is written. It is of no use watching the sick if you have not learnt, or are not learning, the signs that are written in the plainest language for those that have " eyes to see."

I am very appreciative of the kind attention you have paid throughout these lectures to all that I have had to say to you. If they serve to show that I am not ignorant of, nor unsympathetic with, your difficulties, and to convince you of the cordial interest I have in all that affects you and your work, our time will not have been wasted.

In conclusion, will you let me urge upon you, as I did three months ago, to-keep steadily before you a very high standard of the work you have chosen ? I want you to realize how much, how very much, the " tone " of the whole nursing staff depends upon each individual member of it; and then you can decide, individually and collectively, if you mean to rest contented with attaining anything short of the very best. Think of the enormous power you exercise over each other by your daily example. The influence of those in authority is simply nothing in comparison with it. We all feel the effect of public opinion more or less, and the majority of people, if not all, are most influenced by that section of the public, be it large or small, with which they are immediately

concerned. It is, so to speak, the mental atmosphere with
which we are surrounded, and as we were speaking just now
of the air we breathe, and the effect which its condition produces upon us, and the effect which every *one* produces upon
its condition, is it not a matter of vital importance to keep
this mental atmosphere pure and invigorating ? Do you see
what a difference it makes, metaphorically speaking, whether
you are contributing your share of oxygen, or more than your
share of carbonic acid ? When we enter a room too heavily
laden with this noxious gas, we cannot trace the individual
share that each one has had in producing this condition of the
atmosphere; we can only judge of the result. Thus it is with
what I am now speaking of as the mental atmosphere of this
little community. What will be the feeling of those who
enter it from outside ? Will their sensation on entering be,
" This place is stifling ; I wish I had never come in ? " or will
they be conscious of a strong under-current of earnestness
pervading the whole, and gradually driving out the denser
fumes of self-concentration, frivolity, and indifference, which
are apt to become so suffocating, and the influence of which is
likely to have such an insidious effect upon us before we are
aware of it ? If one of your number deteriorates instead of
improves, should it not be a question for each of you to ask
yourselves seriously if you have done your share in preventing
an occurrence which reflects sadly upon the whole ? Dismiss
wholly from your minds the notion that any one of you is too
insignificant for it to matter what you do or say. There is
nothing truer than the fact that while we live at all, it is
impossible to benefit or to injure ourselves only. The whole
human race is bound together in too close links of brother-
hood for that. In the words of a thoughtful writer, I would
ask you to " take the same pride in your life that a poet does
in making his poem, the painter his picture, the engineer his
bridge and his road. . . . Work on honestly, concentratedly,

steadily at what is nearest your hand, and above your toil, which may appear trivial enough, keep shining the fertilizing warmth and brightness of ennobling thoughts and hopes."

Nursing is work that should develop all that is best and highest and most womanly in you ; and if you find this is not so, be sure there is something wrong in the spirit with which you are doing it. Remember that the profession which you have taken up, from motives as varied, probably, as your individual characters, was of old intrusted to the holiest women, and they did not find themselves the worse for it. Why, then, should you ? Our lives and our work are exactly what we determine to make them. Recognize these obvious truths, and make the most of the great opportunities for usefulness which now surround you on every side. I dwell the more emphatically upon the good you can do to each other, because it is more likely to be overlooked than what you can do for your patients. There is perhaps a tendency to forget that the bravest workers are apt to grow weary at times, and to do less than their best for lack of a little opportune encouragement. No one could give this better or so well as a fellow-worker who happens to be feeling stronger than they are at the moment. Probably you will never have an idea of the service you by word or example have rendered to others ; but you will find that there is a curious response in all human nature to words and acts that have a tendency to raise us above our ordinary level.

" Whene'er a noble deed is wrought,
Whene'er is spoken a noble thought,
Our hearts in glad surprise
To higher levels rise.

" The tidal wave of deeper souls
Into our inmost being rolls,
And lifts us unawares
Out of all meaner cares.

"Honour to those whose words and deeds
Thus help us in our daily needs,
And by their overflow
Raise us from what is low ! " *

And there is but one essential to enable you all to do this, and that is that your work should be earnest and true from its very foundation.

"Beautiful it is to see and understand that no worth known or unknown can die even in this earth," says Carlyle ; "for the working of the good and brave endures literally for ever and cannot die." Nothing else lasts, whatever it may *seem* to do, and it is beyond all things encouraging to you to reflect that no single effort for good can by any possibility be really wasted.

Strive to keep such rules as are given you, not only to the letter but to the spirit, because it is *right* for you to do so, not because you get into trouble if you do not. If you choose by influence and example to make an intensely honourable feeling the guiding spirit of this place, it is perfectly possible for you to do so, and you *only* can do this for yourselves. Discipline can and will be officially maintained, of course ; but that is taking such a low ground for *you*, and is a very poor sort of thing compared to the loyal service which is due from you to the hospital whose credit you have at stake when you have once worn its uniform. ·

There are some amongst you who have come to this work in the hope of finding strength to bear their own troubles by seeking to soothe the sorrow of others. To them I can only say, Persevere in the brave path you have chosen, and never doubt that rest and fresh courage will be your reward. In proportion as you are enabled to forget yourself you will be strong. " There is only one lamp which we can carry in our hand, and which will burn through the darkest night,

* " Santa Filomena," Longfellow's Poems.

and make the light of a home for us in a desert place—it is sympathy with everything that breathes."

You will be very poor when your life is over if you are contented with mere surface work, and prefer to shut your eyes to the deeper meanings of things in which you are constantly taking part. Numbers will come within your influence in the public life that you have now entered upon. Take care that every single one shall be the better for coming in contact with you. Men, and women too, grow sceptical of human goodness and purity and kindness and truth, because they see so little that will stand the test of daily life; they find so much to despise, so little to admire, when they look around. But they will never fail to reverence and respect such women as are worthy to inspire these feelings. Let them find that chance in you. They will thankfully avail themselves of it, and you cannot render men a greater service than by making yourselves *fit* for them to believe in.

There is not one of you that could bear the sight of a fellow-creature starving if you had food to give. Surely I need not remind *you* that "man does not live by bread alone." I have told you before that it is especially a woman's, and still more a nurse's, privilege to "comfort and help the weak-hearted." Strive not to grow weary of your noble task. There is no such word as *fail* to those who are faithful. Besides—

"Others will take patience, labour to their heart and hand
From thy hand and thy heart and thy brave cheer,
And God's grace fructify through *thee* to *all*."

Rest assured that those in authority are desirous of helping you to the utmost of their power, and for myself I simply have no words to tell you with what intense earnestness I wish each one of you success.

PRINTED BY WILLIAM CLOWES AND SONS, LIMITED,
LONDON AND BECCLES.

Printed in the United States
By Bookmasters